Glade B. Curtis MD FACOG is a Fellow of the
American College of Obstetrics and Gynecology, and
is in private practice in Utah in the United States.
His other books include *Your Pregnancy Week by
Week, Your Pregnancy Over 30, Your Pregnancy
Questions and Answers*. He is married and has five
children.

Judith Schuler has worked with Dr. Curtis for over
13 years, as his editor and co-author. They have col-
laborated together on more than six books, all
dealing with pregnancy. Judith Schuler earned a
Master of Science degree and Bachelor of Science
degree from the University of Arizona, in Tucson,
Arizona. Before Ms. Schuler became an editor for
HPBooks, where she first met Dr. Curtis, she taught
at university level in California and Arizona. She
lives in southern Arizona with her son.

D1407826

by the same authors

Your Pregnancy Week by Week
Your Pregnancy Questions and Answers
Your Pregnancy After 30

Your Pregnancy
RECOVERY GUIDE

Glade B. Curtis, MD, OB/GYN
&
Judith Schuler

ELEMENT
Shaftesbury, Dorset • Boston, Massachusetts • Melbourne, Victoria

© Element Books Limited 1999
Text © Glade B. Curtis and Judith Schuler 1999

First published in the USA in 1999 by
Element Books, Inc.
160 North Washington Street
Boston, MA 02114

Published in the UK in 1999 by
Element Books Limited
Shaftesbury, Dorset SP7 8BP

Published in Australia in 1999 by
Element Books and distributed
by Penguin Australia Limited
487 Maroondah Highway, Ringwood,
Victoria 3134

Cover photograph: © Tony Stone Images
Cover design by Slatter-Anderson
Text illustrations by David Fischer
Design by Roger Lightfoot
Typeset by WestKey Limited, Falmouth, Cornwall
Printed and bound in the USA by Courier-Westford Inc

British Library Cataloguing-in-Publication
data available

Library of Congress Cataloging-in-Publication
data available

ISBN 1 86204 395 7

Note from the Publisher
This book is in no way intended to replace, countermand or conflict with the advice
given to you by your own physician. The ultimate decision concerning care should
be made between you and your medical practitioner.

Foreword

Participating in the birth of a new baby is exciting for everyone involved—the new parents, family members and friends. It's also exciting for the medical personnel who have been privileged to care for you and your baby before the birth. To those ends—the care of you and your unborn baby—we have written three other books, all dealing with the pregnancy period: *Your Pregnancy Week by Week*, *Your Pregnancy Questions and Answers* and *Your Pregnancy After 30*.

This book is a new venture, in that we cover the period following your baby's birth. Because this is also an important time in your life, it's a subject we've wanted to address for a long time.

The material we've included in this book is intended to help guide you through the many new experiences awaiting you now that your pregnancy is over and your new baby is here.* We even include information to help you plan future pregnancies. We hope the topics covered will assist you in your pregnancy recovery and the beginning of your new life as a parent.

*Please note that throughout the book, we have used "him" or "her" when referring to your baby; some passages will say "she," while other passages may alternate using "he."

Acknowledgments

There are many people we wish to thank for their help and support during the preparation of this book. Without their understanding and assistance, it would have been much more difficult.

Dr. Glade Curtis—I want to thank my wife, Debbie, for her support throughout this project and for always being there, in both good and hard times. Thanks, too, to my five children, for understanding the time and effort a project like this requires. Without the love and support of my parents, I wouldn't be where I am today. Special thanks also to Megan and Scott Harbertsen for their computer expertise.

Judith Schuler—Thanks to my son, Ian, for his understanding and acceptance of all my time and traveling during this project. Thanks too to my Mom and Dad—I greatly appreciate your love and support. Also, my deepest gratitude to Bob Rucinski for his help with my computer. I couldn't have made heads or tails of any of it without your assistance.

Contents

Introduction

The end of labor is a wonderful new beginning. Your beautiful new baby has arrived, and you and your partner are filled with joy, love and happiness that you are now a family. You are busy enjoying your new baby and the attention of your family and friends. You are also probably anxious to get on with the role of parenting this new addition to your family life. However, the first 6 weeks immediately after your baby's birth, called the *postpartum period*, is one of great adjustment, and you probably have many questions and concerns during this exciting new facet of your life.

The Postpartum Period—Your Questions

Some of the many questions you may be asking at this time are as follows.

- How long it will take me to get back on my feet and to recover fully?
- What are the different ways to feed my baby?
- How can I get my body back in shape through exercise and a nutritious eating plan?
- How can I take care of my baby, and not neglect my spouse in this time of adjustment for us both?
- What about returning to work and finding a caregiver?

All of these questions and concerns, as well as many others, are addressed in this book. You may choose to read all the information here, or you may want to check out the sections or chapters that are of most interest to you right now.

CHAPTER 1

The Postpartum Period

The recovery period immediately after your baby's birth (the first 6 weeks) is called the *postpartum period*. Your body undergoes major, rapid shrinking during this time as it begins to return to its prepregnancy size. During the postpartum period, you will go through great physical and emotional adjustments, but this does not mean you are ill—your body is simply re-adapting itself.

You need to take good care of yourself to get back in shape, physically and mentally, and to be ready to face the challenges ahead. Be willing to allow others to help you, and accept the fact you are going to have to take it easy for a while. The time you spend in the hospital after delivery can be very helpful to you in learning how to breastfeed, learning how to take care of the baby and learning how to deal with all the various things happening to you. Most hospitals or delivery suites have educational channels or videotapes on many subjects, such as nursing and childcare, that you can watch while you are in the hospital. Try to learn as much as you can about what to expect after delivery—listen to and follow the advice of your doctor and the nurses at the hospital.

Immediately Following the Birth

Your body has undergone some tremendous changes. Immediately after birth, your uterus begins shrinking rapidly in an effort to control bleeding and to return to its normal prepregnancy state. You will experience pains, called *afterpains*, as your uterus contracts (see p. 3 and p. 25). While your hormone levels are returning to normal, your emotions may fluctuate. You may find you are a little woozy the first few times you get out of bed. Your body may feel stiff and sore from the delivery, and your back may ache. If you had a C-section (Cesarean delivery), your abdominal muscles may be very sore, and you may not be able to get around very quickly. Your body may retain fluid. You may find yourself perspiring more. The good news is that these are all temporary changes! Quite soon, you'll find you have returned to your normal physical state, and each of these changes will soon be merely a memory.

Below are more in-depth discussions about the particular experiences you may have.

Some Changes You May Experience

Bleeding after Delivery
As you pass beyond the time of the birth, one of the many bodily changes you will experience is a discharge of blood, called *lochia*. This occurs as the lining of the uterus is shed; the discharge gradually turns from bright red to pink or brown; and finally to yellow or white before it stops. It is heavy at first but becomes lighter with time. This bleeding will occur whether you had a vaginal delivery or a Cesarean delivery, although it is not quite as heavy with a C-section. It should stop altogether by the time you go for your 6-week postpartum checkup. It should not cause you any concern unless the bleeding suddenly becomes heavy again or if you begin to pass blood clots larger than a silver dollar. If either occurs, call your doctor immediately. (See Chapter 3 for a further discussion of heavy bleeding.)

Perineum Pain
You may have some pain in the perineum, the area between the vagina and the rectum. This is caused by stretching, tearing or cutting of the area to allow for delivery of the baby. During delivery, a controlled cut, called an *episiotomy*, may be made. The pain around the area where this incision was made may be very uncomfortable, but it heals very quickly, and you can take measures to help you feel

more comfortable. For example, you can soak the area by taking sitz baths (a chair-like tub for soaking your lower body and thighs) or take pain medication as prescribed by your doctor. (See Chapter 3 for a further discussion of this type of pain.)

Afterpains
The painful contractions of your uterus known as *afterpains* may occur for several days after your baby is born; these signal that the uterus is shrinking to its prepregnancy size (or as close as it will come to it). You may notice the same type of discomfort when you breastfeed; when you nurse, your body releases a hormone called *oxytocin*, which causes the uterus to contract and your milk to flow. Applying warm compresses to your abdomen, lying for a short time on a warm (but not hot) heating pad and taking oral pain medication can help. (Pain medication is OK to use, even if you are breastfeeding.) (See Chapter 3 for a further discussion of afterpains.)

Pain from Engorged Breasts
Your breasts may feel sore and tender, whether you are breastfeeding or not—you can't stop the natural flow of milk to your breasts, even if you do not plan to nurse your baby. In the past, medication was given to dry up breast milk; this is no longer done because of safety concerns. If you don't breastfeed, the discomfort of engorgement—the fullness in your breasts caused by breast milk—lasts for only a few days. Wear a supportive bra, or bind your breasts tightly with a towel or bandage to ease the pain. Ice packs numb the area and help dry up the milk flow. Do not stimulate your breasts by rubbing the nipples, and avoid running warm water over the area, as this also causes stimulation. Take oral pain medication as prescribed if the pain is severe.

If you decide to breastfeed your baby, you will experience similar discomfort. However, in this case, you will want to stimulate your breasts so that milk production will begin in earnest. You can ease the pain of engorgement by encouraging your baby to breastfeed often. The more often (and longer) she nurses, the sooner your milk production will become established. If your breasts are painfully engorged, and your baby doesn't need to feed again, you can empty your breasts by *expressing* or releasing your milk by hand or with a breast pump. Save any milk you express to feed your baby with another time. (See the discussion of saving breast milk in Chapter 4.)

Your Nutritional Needs

You may be surprised how ravenous you will feel if you are breastfeeding. A breastfeeding mother must produce milk for her nursing infant; nursing takes a lot from your body. It is essential to have good nutrition for this important task, and your hunger ensures that you receive the nutrition you need. If you breastfeed, the nutrients your baby receives depend on the quality of the food you eat. Breastfeeding places more demands on your body than pregnancy. Your body burns up to 1,000 calories a day just to produce milk. When breastfeeding, you need to eat an extra 500 calories a day. Be sure to keep your fluid levels up.

Whatever you do, do *not* attempt to diet at this point! Adequate nutrition will help you recover after the taxing experience of 9 months of pregnancy and the birth of your baby. Be good to yourself—eat the foods that will help you recover and that provide you with the energy you need. Avoid junk food or empty-calorie foods, and drink plenty of fluid, particularly water. (See Chapter 5 for a further discussion of nutrition.)

Exercise is Important for You

Exercise is important to your total feeling of well-being. You can begin doing very light exercises, for example, stretching your muscles and doing Kegel exercises (see p. 67), while you are still in the hospital. Walking around the hospital as soon as you are able is a good exercise. However, before you start any postpartum exercise program, be sure to check with your doctor. He or she may have some particular advice for you. (See Chapter 6, "Exercise After Pregnancy," for a further discussion.)

You will probably be told to be careful with your activity if you had a Cesarean delivery. You need to be cautious about lifting objects and carrying heavy things after a C-Section, which can be difficult, especially if you have other children at home. Avoid any activities that may strain your abdominal muscles. These muscles are not cut during a Cesarean delivery; they are "separated," then sewn together. Because of this condition, bending or stretching can pull or strain the muscles, making you uncomfortable. Take care of your incision, as you have been shown how to do in the hospital. Although infections do not commonly occur, if you have one, it will usually appear 4 to 6 days after the birth.

Other Conditions You May Experience

Constipation, uncomfortable bowel movements and hemorrhoids may be another legacy resulting from the birth. The process of delivery can slow the movement of food through the intestines, which may cause you to feel bloated or constipated. You may also have been given an enema during labor. Changing your diet, taking pain medicine and spending more time in bed all contribute to a condition in which the bowel does not function normally.

When you do have a bowel movement, it is important not to strain. Straining can aggravate hemorrhoids and may cause problems with your episiotomy incision. Drinking plenty of fluids, adding bran and prunes to your diet, and taking stool softeners as recommended by your doctor can help resolve these conditions.

You might experience incontinence (reduced ability to control your flow of urine) for a short period. It's not uncommon for this to occur. Empty your bladder frequently, and do your Kegel exercises (see p. 67) to combat incontinence. As your bladder muscles contract and grow stronger, the incontinence will pass.

You may be very emotional at times following the birth of your baby. You may feel sad, and be confused by your feelings. Nearly 80% of all women who have a baby experience emotional mood swings, called "baby blues." Most often, these mood swings are mild, but some women experience more-severe feelings—this is called *postpartum depression*. (For a thorough discussion of baby blues and the condition of postpartum distress syndrome, see Chapter 3.)

Other emotions you may feel include elation, feelings of inadequacy and feeling overwhelmed by your new responsibilities. You may feel ignored or "out of the limelight." During your pregnancy, a great deal of attention was focused on you; now the focus has shifted to your baby. Some new mothers are surprised and confused when they feel ignored after their baby arrives. It's OK to feel like this; the feeling will soon pass as you become more attached to your baby.

After-Pregnancy Changes

The changes discussed in this section may not happen immediately. However, it's important to include them so you will know what to expect. If you are prepared for these changes, you won't be surprised or upset when they occur.

Abdominal Changes

After the birth of your baby, you may notice changes in your abdominal shape and the skin over the abdomen. Your breast size and shape may also be affected by pregnancy, sometimes permanently.

Some women's abdomens return to normal naturally, but some never return to their prepregnancy state. Abdominal skin is not like muscle, so it can't be strengthened by exercise. One of the main factors that affects your skin's ability to return to its prepregnancy tightness is connective tissue, which provides suppleness and elasticity. As you get older, your skin loses connective tissue and elasticity. Other factors include your state of fitness before you became pregnant, heredity and how greatly your skin was stretched during pregnancy.

Changes in Your Hair

One of the most noticeable changes you may see is in your hair. The hair of many pregnant women enters a growing stage due to increased amounts of estrogen in the body. Usually within 3 months of the baby's birth, a woman's estrogen level decreases, and her hair is affected. It enters a "shedding" phase, where lots of hair falls out. If this happens to you, you are not going bald! As a matter of fact, you will probably end up with about the same amount of hair as you had before you got pregnant—you just seem to be losing a lot of hair now. You may also have experienced a darkening of your hair color during pregnancy if your natural hair color is blond or light brunette. This color change may be permanent.

Changes in Your Skin

Your skin may also have gone through many changes during pregnancy. You may have developed acne, even if you never had it before. It's just another way your body reacted to fluctuating hormones, and your skin should begin to clear up now. However, you may develop acne after your baby is born. If this occurs, over-the-counter topical medication can help. If you're not breastfeeding, your doctor may prescribe a particular medication for you.

Freckles and moles may have darkened and enlarged during pregnancy. You may have also noticed a dark pigment, called *chloasma* or the *mask of pregnancy*, around your nose, cheekbones, forehead, upper lip and eyes. This discoloration usually fades somewhat within 6 months after delivery. Some preparations can be used to help fade the discoloration if you are not breastfeeding—check with your doctor. Skin tags may also have appeared during pregnancy or may appear after birth. These small growths of skin are easily removed by a physician.

Stretch marks are the scars left where your skin stretched, due to your enlarging abdomen and weight gain during pregnancy. Some women have relatively few stretch marks from pregnancy, but others have severe stretch marks. These are caused by weight gain and hormones that allow the skin's elastic fibers to relax and stretch. The stretch marks are probably a purplish-red at this time, but they will gradually fade to silver-white lines within a year or so. Several methods are being experimented with to help avoid or to remove stretch marks, and it is possible that laser treatments may be helpful in the future.

You may notice a change in the coloration of the *areola*, the area around the nipple. It may darken and enlarge slightly. Researchers believe this occurs as a signal to the breastfeeding infant. Discoloration usually lightens within a few months after the birth, although the areolas may remain darker than they were before pregnancy.

If the *linea nigra*—the dark line of pigmentation that runs from your bellybutton down to the pubis symphysis—darkened on your body, it will fade after a few months, but it may never disappear. Not all pregnant women have it, but if you do, there is nothing harmful about it.

Changes in Your Teeth and Sense of Smell

Some women find that their sense of smell is more acute during pregnancy. This usually begins to fade 6 to 8 weeks after the birth. If your gums bled more easily during pregnancy, the condition should begin to correct itself. Keep flossing and brushing your teeth regularly. You might want to schedule a dental cleaning and an exam now that your baby is here, as it is important that your teeth are in good condition.

Swelling of Your Limbs and Nail Changes

If you experienced swelling in your legs, hands or feet during pregnancy, this will lessen or disappear within a couple of weeks. Most women find that their feet spread and their shoe size increases by at least one-half size—this may be a permanent change. Varicose veins (see p. 29) may disappear, but spider veins could be permanent. If your fingernails and toenails grew rapidly while you were pregnant, the growth will probably slow down to a normal rate within a couple of weeks of the birth. Your nails may become brittle after your baby's birth.

Bonding with Your Baby

You've probably heard how important it is to "bond with your baby." What is bonding? Is it that important in your new life with your baby? When does it happen? And how does it happen?

Bonding is not necessarily immediate—it's a process and can take longer than one instance to occur. It's the feeling of being emotionally attached to your child, which deepens with time. Bonding occurs separately between each parent and his or her child. We once believed bonding was purely an emotional response; today researchers know there is also a physical aspect to bonding. Bonding stimulates the production of the hormones prolactin and oxytocin in the mother; in fact, it is now believed that these hormones help a woman to have a "mothering" feeling toward her infant. The bonding process also helps keep the baby's hormones in balance.

A mother can bond with her child at different times and during different stages of their relationship. You can bond with your baby the first time in the delivery room, your hospital room or even at home. Don't be afraid that the bond will be weaker if you cannot "meet" in the delivery room.

Some feel that bonding begins before birth, while the baby is still inside the uterus. Bonding during pregnancy can involve either or both parents. (See Chapter 8, pp. 99–100, for a further discussion of bonding for both the new father and mother).

However, the hour following birth is usually the prime bonding time for mom, dad and baby. Mother and infant are programmed to connect at this time. Both need each other. The woman needs to see, touch, smell and hold this person she has carried for 9 months. The baby needs the comfort of its mother's touch after going through the birth process.

Sometimes bonding begins in the delivery room. Ask if procedures normally done can safely be postponed for a little while to facilitate bonding at this stage. If you can't hold your baby, ask your partner or a nurse to hold the baby up to your face, where you can nuzzle him with your cheek. Bonding can continue in your hospital room, if your hospital allows "rooming in." You can respond to your baby as soon as he begins to cry or make noises.

Nursing is one of the best ways to bond with your baby, especially if you are feeding her on demand. This enables you to respond to your baby whenever she needs you. Don't despair if you do not breastfeed; you can achieve the same degree of bonding when bottlefeeding by responding to your baby whenever she cries. Look at her, talk to her and hold her close. Create as much skin-to-skin contact as possible. As your infant begins to mature, this bonding process will be strengthened—just relax and let it happen.

Dads can bond with baby, too. Invite your partner to be part of the bonding process by encouraging him to hold the baby close, like you do, while making eye and skin contact. He can respond just as you do to the baby's cries. You may ask him to feed the baby when you begin expressing your breast milk.

The key to bonding is to focus on the baby and the experiences you share. Holding and cuddling your baby, or cooing to her, are great ways to bond. No matter when the bonding actually occurs, your baby will connect with you because she will feel the love and security you are giving her.

Examinations Following Delivery

Most doctors will want you to come in to see them for an exam following a C-section or postpartum tubal ligation 10 to 14 days after you leave the hospital. The doctor will want to examine the incision to see if it is healing properly and to look for any signs of infection, such as redness or leakage of fluid or pus from the incision. A pelvic exam is not usually done at this visit.

The doctor will ask if you are having problems, such as bleeding, pain, problems with breastfeeding or difficulty with bowel movements or bladder function. If you were anemic after delivery, you may need to have a blood test. Before you leave the office, make an appointment for your 6-week checkup, if you haven't done so already.

The 6-week postpartum checkup is an important visit; make sure you keep this appointment. A pelvic exam done at this checkup ensures that your uterus is getting smaller and that there are no blood clots or tissue left inside. If you have had an episiotomy, it will be checked at this time.

The Postpartum Checkup

Your body will change greatly during the next 4 to 6 weeks. By the time you visit your doctor for your 6-week postpartum checkup, your uterus will have shrunken to the size of a grapefruit. That's an incredible feat, considering it was the size of a small watermelon only a few short weeks before!

At your postpartum checkup, your doctor will check your weight and blood pressure—in much the same way as at your prenatal appointments. Your doctor will give you a pelvic exam to check your vagina, uterus and cervix to see how far healing has progressed. Your breasts may also be checked for size and shape.

If you had a vaginal birth, your doctor will examine any tears or incisions you had. If you had a C-section, your doctor will check that incision. If you developed hemorrhoids or varicose veins during pregnancy, your doctor will want to check those, too.

If you have any questions about your recovery, be sure to address them with your physician at this time. It's also a good time to discuss your birth-control options, as you do not want to become pregnant again immediately. (See Chapter 10 for a further discussion of birth-control options and planning future pregnancies.) Read the following chapter for an in-depth discussion of the recovery period.

CHAPTER 2

After Your Baby's Birth

Having a baby is a rewarding experience, but it is also very draining physically and emotionally. You will probably be very tired when everything is over and may feel emotionally drained. Your stay in the hospital will allow you to relax and regroup before you go home with your baby—take advantage of this time and the resources available to you there. From this time on, you will need to continue taking good care of yourself so that you can heal quickly and get on with taking care of your new baby.

While you are still in the hospital, the nursing staff are available to help you if you have any questions about your care or the care of your baby. Nursing staff are often more knowledgeable than doctors about breastfeeding, and will be happy to help you when you begin. They can also show you how to do the normal things needed to care for your baby, such as bathing or diapering him. They will provide advice about taking care of yourself, such as dealing with your episiotomy and caring for your breasts. They will also allow you to rest—something you probably need very much. If you are very hungry, which is often the case after the hard work of giving birth, it will help to eat a good meal. If you had to watch your weight closely during pregnancy, reward yourself with something that tastes fabulous! Don't go on a strict diet right away—wait awhile. Even if you don't breastfeed your baby, your body requires a well-balanced, nutritious diet for you to stay healthy and to keep your energy levels up. (See Chapter 5, "Nutrition to Get Back in Shape," for a further discussion.)

Most women are discharged within a day or two after their baby's birth, as long as the labor and delivery were normal and the baby is doing well. Whether you had a vaginal or Cesarean delivery, you are monitored closely for the first few hours following the birth and offered medication to relieve pain as necessary. As you recover in your room, your urine output may be checked, to ensure that your kidneys and bladder are working properly. If you had an episiotomy or a Cesarean, nurses will check your incision to make sure it heals properly. They will also monitor your blood pressure, the amount of bleeding and your overall health as you recover.

You will probably experience two main areas of pain—your abdomen and your episiotomy (if you had one). Don't hesitate to ask for pain medication if you are experiencing either abdominal or episiotomy pain.

Tubal Ligation

Some women choose to have a form of surgical sterilization performed, called a *tubal ligation*, while they are in the hospital after their baby's birth. This operation involves tying a woman's tubes to prevent further pregnancies. If you haven't thought seriously about it before, however, this is *not* the time to make a decision about a tubal ligation, as the procedure is usually permanent.

If you have already decided prior to your delivery to have a tubal ligation, it is sensible to do this after your delivery, as you're already in the hospital. If you also received an epidural during your delivery, you would already be anesthetized for the tubal ligation. However, if you didn't have an epidural, in most cases, the tubal ligation procedure requires you to be anesthetized under a general anesthetic.

There are disadvantages to having a tubal ligation immediately after your baby's birth, particularly as this surgery is usually considered permanent and irreversible. If you have your tubes tied within a few hours or a day after having your baby, and then change your mind, you may regret it.

Recovery from a Vaginal Birth

Doctors frequently hear new parents remark in relief, "It's over!" following the delivery of their baby. It's true that the 9 long months of pregnancy and labor and delivery are now over, but another very exciting and perhaps even-more-challenging part of life has just begun!

In the Hospital after a Vaginal Birth
One of the first things you may notice after your delivery is how tired you are. This is true for both vaginal and Cesarean deliveries. Some women have compared the feeling of exhaustion to how a person feels after running a marathon.

As the excitement of the birth settles down, it isn't unusual to be worn out. Allow yourself to rest and to recover while you're in the hospital. Take advantage of the "built-in" room service and baby-sitting provided in the hospital. You probably won't have this luxury when you go home, especially if you have young children.

For the first hour after delivery, the nurses will check you frequently for bleeding, pain, blood-pressure problems and other warning signs while you and your partner bond with your new baby. The baby is also being evaluated. During this time you will probably only be allowed ice chips and sips of water, even though you may be anxious to eat some food and to drink some fluids.

The restriction of food and drink is for your safety; if there are any problems, such as heavy bleeding, it is sometimes necessary to perform minor surgery, such as a dilatation and curettage (D&C), a surgical procedure in which the cervix is dilated and the lining of the uterus is scraped. It is safer for you if your stomach is empty if this operation is necessary.

Dealing with Contractions and Pain after Delivery
You may have thought that once you delivered, the contractions would disappear. Actually it's important for your uterus to contract at this time in order to prevent excessive bleeding. Nursing your baby helps make the contractions stronger.

Another source of discomfort after you deliver will be in your vagina, and between the opening of the vagina and the rectum (the perineum). This is the area where an episiotomy is made or any tearing occurs during delivery, when the baby's head or shoulders begin to emerge. You will be offered pain medicine and ice packs to help with any swelling and pain. Your nurse will teach you how to take care of this area while you are in the hospital and when you go home.

Medicine is available to you to help deal with contractions and pain. Most often it is not given routinely; it is ordered for you, and all you have to do is ask for it. Initially, pain medicine may be given in the form of an injection until you are allowed to drink and eat. After that, you will usually be offered pain pills, such as ibuprofen or acetaminophen (Tylenol®), as well as stronger pain medications, such as Tylenol #3®.

It is normal to bleed after delivery; bleeding continues for anywhere from several days to a couple of weeks. Your nurse will check your bleeding frequently to make sure it is not excessive. It is sometimes difficult to say how much bleeding is too much; your doctor and the nurses will evaluate this. After delivery, the bleeding should gradually slow down, but you will still be bleeding when you go home from the hospital. Most often, medication is given to you at the time of delivery, either by an I.V. or injection, to help your uterus contract and prevent excessive bleeding.

If there is any possibility of infection after delivery, you may be given antibiotics while in the hospital. If your bleeding is excessive, you may be given vitamins and iron supplements to combat blood loss. If you are Rh-negative, you may be given RhoGAM®.

Passing urine may be uncomfortable or may hurt. This usually doesn't last very long, and does not necessarily mean that you have a bladder or urinary-tract infection (UTI). Just take it easy, and take your time when you have to go to the bathroom.

Having your first bowel movement may be an adventure. Laxatives or stool softeners are often given while you are in the hospital so you don't become constipated. If you had an enema at the beginning of labor, this can help lessen the problem of a painful bowel movement after delivery.

Dealing with Visitors
Your friends and family will want to visit you while you are recovering in the hospital. This can be very enjoyable for everyone and can be a very valuable time for both you and for them. However, don't be afraid to limit the time spent with visitors—either in person or on the telephone. There is nothing wrong with putting a hold on your phone calls or a "Do not disturb" sign on your door when you want to rest.

Ask your visitors to check with the nurses before coming into your room. Most people are very understanding about this, particularly if they have children of their own.

When You Go Home
Before you leave the hospital, your doctor and pediatrician will talk to you about when you or your baby need to see them for a checkup.

When you go home, you will still be bleeding, but the amount of bloody discharge you pass should be decreasing. Sometimes when you go home and are more active, the bleeding may be a little heavier at first, but this shouldn't last more than a few hours before it slows down again.

It is normal to have cramps and/or pain in the area of the episiotomy when you go home. This should lessen every day. Usually you will be given a prescription for mild pain medications when you go home. It's OK to take these medicines, but usually they will not be needed as often once you are home.

Fatigue and exhaustion may become more of a problem. Now you have to do it all yourself—no nurses or hospital staff are there to help you out! Don't be afraid to ask for help, and do allow people to help you. Most people are anxious to do this and also enjoy it. Your partner will want to help, but he may not know what to do. He may appreciate suggestions from you about how he can help, such as getting up in the middle of the night to feed the baby (if bottlefeeding) or bringing her to you to nurse.

Besides pain medicines, you may want to continue to take prenatal vitamins or iron once you go home. Many doctors will encourage you to continue taking stool softeners or laxatives, for the reasons already discussed (see p. 14).

Activities after a Vaginal Birth
Your main activity immediately after delivery will be trying to keep up with your new baby and his many needs. You also have to think about your own needs in recovering after labor and delivery.

If you have had an epidural, it takes a few hours for it to wear off before you are able to get out of bed. However, within a few hours you'll be able to get out of bed and walk around or go to the bathroom. Don't try to do too much or worry about exercising. Most doctors suggest that you not just sit in bed (we often describe this as "sitting in bed watching TV, eating bon-bons and taking pain pills"); it's usually better to get out of bed and go for a walk, but be careful not to push it at this time.

When you go home, gradually increase your activities. You can walk around, eat more normally and gradually become more active each day. You may also feel like you need to rest frequently—that's OK. Pay attention to your own body as to what you feel up to doing.

Most doctors recommend that you come in for a 6-week postpartum checkup before you begin any strenuous activity or exercise, or become sexually active again. See the discussion in Chapter 10.

Many women ask about driving and going up and down stairs. If you're still taking pain medicines or are experiencing any dizziness, don't drive. It's OK to use the stairs, but it's wise to plan ahead so that you are not running up and down stairs all day. Park yourself where you are comfortable, are close to the baby, and have food and beverages near at hand.

Precautions after a Vaginal Birth

The nurses and your doctor will go over any warning signs and precautions with you before you go home. This includes instructions about normal bleeding and what to do about pain. If you have any problems, it's helpful when you call your doctor to give him or her information about bleeding, such as how many pads you are using, if there are clots and what you have done or taken to help deal with the problem. See the list on pp. 23–4.

If you start to exercise and experience any problems, such as heavy bleeding, pain or dizziness, talk to your doctor before continuing an exercise program.

Most physicians suggest that you not have sexual intercourse until after you have had your 6-week postpartum checkup. Even at 6 weeks, you may not be ready if your episiotomy is still sore or if you are still bleeding.

How Long Until You're Back on Your Feet?

Full recovery is different for every woman, but there are some basic guidelines. These are general guidelines; if you have had complications or problems, it may be different for you.

Following a normal pregnancy and delivery, most doctors suggest that you come to see them 6 weeks after delivery for a postpartum checkup. This 6-week visit is a good time to talk to your doctor about contraception. At this point, it is usually OK to resume routine activities, such as exercise, intercourse or returning to work. If you have experienced problems or complications, be sure to ask your doctor about them before resuming activities. If you are returning to work, make plans weeks before you return for childcare, nursing, your own recovery and whether you are going to work full-time or part-time (see Chapter 9 for a further discussion of preparing to return to work).

Taking Care of Your Baby
For 6 or 7 months, you saw your doctor regularly to monitor the progress of your pregnancy. After delivery, you are no longer the center of attention—your baby is!

In the first 24 hours after delivery, you and your baby will probably still be in the hospital. Your baby's pediatrician will come to the hospital, do a physical on the baby, then see you to arrange an appointment for your baby. If you had a boy, the pediatrician will talk to you about your preferences regarding circumcision. Your signature is required before this can be done. In some areas, your obstetrician will do this, while in other areas, it is performed by the pediatrician or family practitioner.

During the first 24 hours, much of your time is spent getting to know your baby. You thought it was difficult to sleep at night during the pregnancy because you were uncomfortable—at least then you didn't have to feed anyone or change their diapers! Personnel at the hospital evaluate you and your baby to make sure you are both doing OK and can safely go home.

The first week after birth, you will probably try to get some kind of schedule for you and your baby. Don't be surprised if the baby isn't conforming to your plans; this can take weeks or months.

During this first week, try to nap or rest whenever you can. When your baby sleeps, it's a good time for you to rest also. Try to avoid the temptation to catch up on your housework.

From 2 to 6 weeks, you should be feeling a little better every day. At this point, you probably won't be taking pain medicine any longer, and the bleeding will be decreasing or gone. You will still have a full-time job taking care of your newborn, but you should be able to find some time for yourself and for your partner. Other than going for your 6-week postpartum checkup with your doctor, your time will be spent more with the pediatrician for routine visits or problems with your newborn.

The first 6 months after delivery consist of a lot of hard work. It is a challenging time but also a very enjoyable and rewarding one as your baby grows and starts to respond to you and to your partner. If you work outside of the home, you will soon be getting back to work. If you exercise, each week you should see results, and you may even find that it is possible that you will get your figure back.

By the end of the first year after delivery, you will have this "baby thing" down. A sure sign of this is that you may even be talking about another pregnancy. During the first year, you spend a lot of time and energy caring for your baby, but gradually during this time you should be able to find time for yourself. This may take some effort; you may want to trade tending time with another new mom on a regular basis so that you will have time for other things.

Recovery from a Cesarean Delivery

There are many similarities in recovering from a vaginal delivery and a Cesarean delivery. However, there are some distinct differences. I have often asked women who have had both a Cesarean delivery and a vaginal delivery which they prefer. I've found it interesting to hear the reasons why some prefer one or the other. There are those who definitely prefer a C-section, and others who definitely prefer a vaginal delivery!

In the Hospital
Immediately after your C-section, you are taken to a recovery room or recovery area for about an hour. Here you are watched for any signs of problems, such as bleeding or pain. Your blood pressure and other vital signs, such as your pulse and temperature, are checked frequently. At this same time, your baby may go to the nursery to be weighed and evaluated, but he is usually returned to you in the recovery room. This is a good time to begin nursing your baby. When you leave the recovery area, you will go to a room where you will spend the remainder of your time in the hospital.

How long a woman stays in the hospital after a Cesarean delivery varies quite a bit. Most women stay for 2 to 4 days after the delivery; an average stay would be 3 days after a C-section. Your insurance or HMO has the greatest say about this, not you or your doctor.

It is normal to bleed vaginally after a Cesarean; this will continue for several days, even up to a few weeks. However, it should decrease each day. The nurses will check to see it is not excessive and will instruct you what to look for after you go home.

Cramping and contraction of your uterus are normal and desirable after a C-section. Contractions of the uterus help control and decrease bleeding after your delivery. With a C-section, there is pain from the surgery itself, but at least you won't have episiotomy pain.

Pain control after a Cesarean is accomplished in different ways. If you had an epidural or spinal anesthetic for the surgery, you may be able to have pain medicine injected through the epidural or spinal catheter; this is called *Duramorph* or *epidural morphine*. This medication usually offers pain relief for the first 24 hours and helps you to avoid further painful injections or pain pills on the first day after surgery.

Other choices for pain relief are those traditionally used following surgery, such as injections of pain medications (Demerol® or morphine) into an I.V. or into a muscle, or other pain medications given during the first 24 hours after delivery until you are able to eat. Once you are able to eat, you may be offered oral pain medications, such as mild narcotics (Tylenol #3® or Lortab®) or anti-inflammatory pain medications, such as ibuprofen.

If you were in labor for a long time before delivery, you may be exhausted. Time spent in the hospital should be an opportunity for you to get some rest and to get ready for the challenges awaiting you at home. Don't be afraid to accept help or suggestions from the nurses or others at the hospital. There are specific areas the nurses at the hospital can help you with and teach you about, such as nursing, caring for your baby and the warning signs of various problems you may encounter after you go home.

In most cases with a C-section, a catheter is placed in your bladder through the urethra (the small tube from the bladder to the outside) before starting the surgery to keep the bladder out of the way during surgery. The catheter is usually left in place for 12 to 24 hours after the surgery. It is a good idea to discuss this with your doctor, as different doctors have different methods of handling this.

Problems with gas or bowel movements are more likely following a C-section than with a vaginal delivery, but there are things you can do to minimize them. Get up and walk around as soon as possible. You may need help with this at first. Drink plenty of liquids; this is more important than trying to eat solid foods in the first few days after delivery. Sitting in bed and/or taking pain medications, vitamins or iron can all cause changes or problems with your bowels. The sooner you get moving, stop taking pain medications and start eating a more-normal diet, the sooner your bowels will return to normal. Laxatives or stool softeners are available if necessary. Although it may seem unpleasant, passing gas is a good sign that your bowels are working.

The doctor and nurses will check your C-section incision daily for infection or bleeding while you are in the hospital. If staples were used on the incision, they are usually removed before you leave the hospital on the second or third post-operative day. This may seem a little soon, but don't worry; the layers of tissue that actually hold you together are deeper. If sutures were used to close the skin, they may have to be removed. Sutures will dissolve on their own, but that may take weeks or even months. Most doctors place steri-strips (like small pieces of tape) on the incision; these stay on for 3 or 4 days. Before you leave the hospital, the nurses will show you how to take care of the incision and will advise you of any warning signs you may need to watch out for when you go home.

When You Go Home
When you go home from the hospital, you will be eating, drinking and walking. Your incision is likely to be sore, and you will still be bleeding vaginally. Most women will still need to take mild pain medication after they go home; you will be offered prescriptions for this before you leave the hospital. Sometimes pain or bleeding increase after you go home and increase your activities. However, you should see an overall decrease in pain and bleeding every day.

Your doctor will recommend that you do not drive if you are taking pain medicine or have other problems, such as anemia. You may not want to drive for a few weeks, particularly if you are uncomfortable or have trouble getting in or out of your car.

Activities after a Cesarean Section
It's OK to increase your activity, but try not to be in too big a hurry. Friends and family are usually more than happy to help out; let them! It is wise to plan your activities to save your energy to take care of yourself and your baby. This includes stairs—plan ahead! If you are

running up and down the stairs all day, chances are you will tire more easily and experience more pain.

Certain activities may not be a good idea because of increased pain, or they may cause complications that could slow down your recovery. During the first few weeks, don't lift anything heavier than your baby. Vacuuming probably isn't going to be harmful, but it may cause you pain because of the stretching or pulling.

It is too soon in the first few weeks to start exercising or resume sexual relations. Most doctors will want to see you in the office 10 to 14 days after your C-section to check your incision and see how you are doing. This visit is a good time to ask how soon you can safely resume activities and what levels of exercise are appropriate.

Precautions after a C-Section

Most doctors suggest that you don't have sexual relations until after your 6-week postpartum visit. In most cases, you won't be ready for relations prior to this time because you are still bleeding, in pain or fatigued. Resuming relations too soon can be harmful because of the risk of possible infection or increased bleeding and can actually delay your recovery.

It is also wise to wait to resume exercising until after your doctor gives you the go ahead. Most doctors will want to see you 6 weeks after the C-section, and if you are doing well at this stage they will clear you for exercise.

Most hospitals and doctors will explain what warning signs to be alert for, such as pain, bleeding, fever or signs of infection. If you feel that something is not right, call your doctor—he expects this and can refer you to specific people to help you with problems. Part of the reason it is essential to go to your appointments before you deliver is to get to know the people there so that you will be comfortable asking them questions both before and after the birth. Other good sources of information include the nurses in the birthing center or hospital where you delivered, or the emergency room. Most area hospitals have nurses available 24 hours a day that you can call for advice.

Getting Back on Your Feet

The rate of recovery is different for every woman. Usually you can return to your normal activities after your 6-week checkup if you are not having problems. Be prepared to ease back into things slowly, and don't expect to pick up immediately where you left off. A C-section is a major surgery, which requires a painful abdominal incision. Besides the normal recovery from surgery, you will also have a 24-hour full-time job taking care of your baby!

When you go home from the hospital, you will be able to get in and out of bed on your own and walk around. Certain activities, such as bending or lifting, may be uncomfortable; take these things slowly at first. Once again, your overall recovery will be smoother if you take care of yourself, rest when necessary and increase your activities gradually.

Taking Care of Your Baby

Most new parents feel overwhelmed and inadequate with their new responsibility. Be assured that you will do great, and will learn as you go! There are many ways to get help and advice—from friends, family, your pediatrician's office and even people you meet in the hospital. Caring for your baby after a C-section should be the same as caring for your baby following a vaginal delivery.

In the first 48 hours following your C-section, you are recovering from the surgery. You will begin eating and moving around. You will also be learning a lot about caring for your baby and what to watch out for in your own recovery.

As the first week progresses, you will be trying to establish a routine for feeding, sleeping and caring for your baby.

From week 2 to week 6, you will notice gradual improvements in your energy every day. After 6 weeks, you should be able to do anything you want. In the months to come, there may not be big changes, but you will notice more-subtle improvements.

CHAPTER 3

Concerns You May Have
During the Recovery Period

You've just had your baby, and everything is great . . . isn't it?

You can probably answer "yes" to that question, but you may have a few concerns about your postpartum recovery period. These concerns are normal—nearly every woman wonders about some of them—just as your "problems" are also normal, whether these are physical or emotional.

You may want to read about all the various topics in this chapter, or you may want to read only about those you are interested in. We have tried to give you the information you need so that you may be reassured that what you are experiencing is not unusual. If you have questions about any of this information or if you are concerned about your particular situation, call your doctor. He or she is there to answer your questions and to offer you reassurance.

Some Warning Signs

Normally, your recovery should go well after your baby's birth—you shouldn't feel ill. However, you might occasionally experience a problem. Below is a list of symptoms and warnings signs to be on the alert for:

- a temperature of 101°F (38.3°C) or more, except in the first 24 hours after birth

- painful or red breasts
- chills
- loss of appetite for an extended period
- pain in the lower abdomen or back
- pain, tenderness, redness and/or swelling in your legs
- painful urination or feeling an intense need to urinate
- failure to pass gas or severe constipation (no bowel movements for a few days)
- severe pain in the vagina or perineum (the area between the rectum and the vagina)
- unusually heavy bleeding or a sudden increase in bleeding (more than your normal menstrual flow at its heaviest, such as soaking more than two sanitary pads in 30 minutes)
- a vaginal discharge with a strong, unpleasant odor

If you experience any of the above symptoms, call your doctor. It's important information to share with him or her. Your doctor may want to see you and prescribe a course of treatment for you.

Concerns for Mothers Who Had Special Problems during Pregnancy

If you have a chronic illness, such as diabetes or gestational diabetes (worsening of or occurrence of diabetes during pregnancy), it may have an impact on your postpartum recovery. You may need to watch for specific problems or make particular adjustments. For example, you may need to eat more food or eat more often than usual if you are breastfeeding. Your insulin requirements may also change, and you may need to monitor your blood sugar more closely.

If you had gestational diabetes during pregnancy, you may need to have your blood-sugar levels tested after delivery. Discuss this with your doctor at your 6-week checkup. If your blood-sugar level is normal, you're OK. If it isn't, you may be referred to a doctor who specializes in treating diabetes. He or she can help you plan a program to deal with your problem. Usually gestational diabetes is cured by delivery, and it does not recur until you are pregnant again.

Changes in the Uterus

After your baby is born, your uterus goes through great changes before returning to its original shape. Just before birth, your uterus is large enough to accommodate the baby; after the birth, it begins to shrink by a finger's width daily, a process known as *involution*. Immediately after delivery, you should be able to feel your uterus around your navel, and it should be quite hard. If it feels soft, you or a nurse can massage it so that it becomes firm. You will be checked daily while you are still in the hospital to ensure that your uterus is shrinking normally and remains hard. This exam may cause some discomfort.

Afterpains

Afterpains are just what they sound like—the pains you experience after the birth of your baby. They are normal, and you should expect to feel them for several days after birth while your uterus contracts. This occurs to prevent heavy bleeding and enable the uterus to return to its normal size. You can ease your cramps by lying on your stomach and by taking mild pain relievers. Drinking lots of fluid so that you urinate often and empty your bladder helps the uterus to work more efficiently and less painfully.

If you're breastfeeding, you may find that your afterpains intensify when you nurse your baby. The baby's sucking stimulates the pituitary gland to release oxytocin, which makes the uterus contract. These extra contractions are good for you, as they help to decrease and control bleeding, but they may be painful. Mild pain medication, such as acetaminophen or ibuprofen, can offer relief.

Perineum Pain

Stretching, cutting or tearing during labor causes pain in the perineum (the area between the vagina and anus). If you had an episiotomy (a surgical incision of the vulva—the area between the vagina and rectum), this can add to your discomfort. However, most perineal soreness should improve daily and is usually gone after 3 weeks or by the time you see your doctor for your 6-week checkup.

If you are experiencing severe discomfort, you may try using ice packs, which offer some relief in the first 24 hours after delivery. Ice numbs the pain and helps reduce swelling. After 24 hours, a warm bath or soaking several times a day in a sitz tub (a chair-type bath, which soaks the thighs and hips) can help.

Other remedies for perineal pain include numbing sprays, witch-hazel compresses, walking to stimulate circulation and practicing your Kegel exercises. Soaking pads in over-the-counter hemorrhoid medication, then freezing them and placing them on the sore area provides excellent relief.

Urinating may be painful as urine can sting the cut area. This pain is not an indication of a urinary-tract infection (UTI) or bladder infection but is merely because of the natural chemicals in the urine that cause the stinging sensation along the cut. You may find it less painful to urinate while standing up or in the shower with running water washing over the area.

Heavy Bleeding after Delivery

It's common to lose blood during labor and delivery, and there is usually some bleeding after delivery. However, you may be concerned if you experience very heavy bleeding after the baby is born. A loss of more than 17 fluid ounces (500ml) in the first 24 hours after delivery is called a *postpartum hemorrhage*.

The most common causes of heavy bleeding after birth include the following:

- when your uterus doesn't contract
- a large or bleeding episiotomy
- a tear, rupture or hole in the uterus (rare)
- clotting or coagulation problems
- a failure of the blood vessels inside the uterus to compress
- retained placental tissue or retained blood clots in the uterus
- rips or tears in the vagina or cervix during birth

Post-delivery bleeding is controlled by massaging the uterus (called *Credé*) and taking certain medications, such as pitocin or methergine. The normal bleeding after delivery, called *lochia*, gradually decreases each day, then stops, although it may become a little heavier as you increase your activities.

If your bleeding suddenly becomes heavy after a few days or weeks, contact your doctor. He or she may want to see you or prescribe medication.

Your Bowel Habits

It's not unusual for your bowel habits to change for a few days after your baby's birth. Your digestive system slows down because of pain medications given to help relieve labor and delivery pain, and because of changes in your activity level or because you are sitting or lying in bed. You may have had an enema, or the lower part of your bowel (the rectum) may have emptied while you pushed during labor and delivery. All of these factors will contribute to bowel-habit changes.

Many women don't want to have to deal with the pain of having a bowel movement for the first 4 or 5 days after delivery. Some new mothers have said that their first bowel movement after the delivery felt like they were delivering another baby.

Bowel Movements after Episiotomies or with Hemorrhoids
If you had an episiotomy or have hemorrhoids, these can make a bowel movement more difficult or more painful, and you may be more apprehensive about it. However, this is not a good time to be constipated. If you want to avoid constipation, eat a high-fiber diet and drink lots of fluid to keep your system working efficiently—prune juice and bran are excellent natural laxatives but over-the-counter stool softeners may also be beneficial. If you don't have a bowel movement within a week, or if you become uncomfortable, contact your doctor.

When you do have a bowel movement, try not to strain. This can aggravate hemorrhoids or make an episiotomy incision or the area of a laceration hurt or bleed.

If you have hemorrhoids after delivery, it's helpful to know that they will eventually shrink on their own, although they probably won't go away completely. A witch-hazel compress or a commercial compress can offer relief. Over-the-counter creams and ointments and mild pain medication or anti-inflammatories, such as ibuprofen, can also offer some relief. Ice packs may also help. More-serious measures are usually unnecessary.

Your Breasts

Whether you breastfeed or bottlefeed, sore breasts are fairly common after delivery. In the natural course of pregnancy and delivery, your body expects you to breastfeed, so your breasts have been preparing through your pregnancy to nurse your baby and will fill with milk.

The fullness of milk in your breasts, called *engorgement*, usually lasts for a few days and can be uncomfortable. If you breastfeed, you can empty your breasts when the baby nurses, and the situation resolves itself in a few days. This situation is a little more difficult for a woman who chooses not to breastfeed, as your milk still comes in; medication is no longer given to dry up this milk. You can ease discomfort by wearing a support bra or binding your breasts with an Ace bandage or a towel. Ice packs also help dry up milk.

If you find your breasts are engorged, and you are not breastfeeding, try *not* to empty your breasts. This may be difficult; emptying your breasts may be the only way to get relief. However, when you empty your breasts, your body replaces the expressed breast milk with more milk! Avoid nipple stimulation and warm water on the breasts because these practices also stimulate your breasts to produce milk. Hearing a baby cry—yours or someone else's—may make you lose milk.

A mild fever with engorgement is not uncommon. Acetaminophen can help with both the fever and the discomfort from engorgement. For further information on problems associated with breastfeeding, such as plugged milk ducts and breast infections, see Chapter 4.

Urinary Incontinence

Bladder function or voiding urine can be very different after delivery for many reasons. During labor and afterward, fluids are often given by I.V. Oxytocin (Pitocin®), given during or after labor, has an "anti-diurectic" effect; it causes a decrease in your urine production. Once this effect has passed, you have a lot of fluid to get rid of—you'll need to urinate a lot! Bladder sensation can also be affected by pain from an episiotomy or a tear in the birth canal, or by anesthesia, such as an epidural.

After a baby is born, some women have trouble controlling their urine; this is called *urinary incontinence*. This may last briefly or may go on for a few weeks or longer. Most women report that the more pregnancies and deliveries they have, the more problems they have with incontinence. There are several factors that contribute to this, including the birth, the size of the baby, the number of deliveries, the size of the uterus and your age.

It is amazing that a baby's head and shoulders can fit through the birth canal. This requires the muscle tissues to stretch a great deal. Your bladder lies in front of the uterus, and the lower part of the bladder wall is stretched during birth. After delivery, this area is weaker than before pregnancy, which may contribute to incontinence.

Each delivery stretches the birth canal. Tissues that support the bladder are also stretched with each delivery, causing some incontinence.

It will take a few weeks or more for your uterus to return to its normal size. In the weeks immediately after delivery, the uterus gradually contracts and grows smaller, but it then presses on the bladder. This compresses it, so your bladder won't hold as much urine, and it might be harder for you to control urine loss.

You can help yourself regain bladder and urine control by practicing Kegel exercises. Try not to hold your urine, and empty your bladder fairly often. Don't expect things to get better immediately—giving birth changes your bladder function; chances are that your bladder control may not be the same as before you became pregnant.

Let your doctor know if a urinary incontinence problem continues or worsens. Improvement may not come for weeks after delivery, once you begin to get back in shape. Surgery may help, but most doctors prefer you to be through having children before this is considered as subsequent pregnancies may undo the effects of the operation involved.

Varicose Veins

Varicose veins (blood vessels that are dilated or enlarged) are a fairly common result of pregnancy. They are also called *varicosities*. You may have an inherited predisposition to varicose veins—if your mother had them, you have a greater chance of having them, too.

Varicose veins occur most often in the legs, but they may also occur in the vulva and vagina. Varicosities will not disappear immediately after delivery. Follow the tips you were given during pregnancy to help deal with varicose veins after your baby is born. Some of these tips include:

- lie on your side (left is best) as much as possible
- elevate your legs above the level of your heart when possible
- don't wear restrictive clothing
- get up and walk when you can
- don't cross your legs
- get regular exercise
- don't stand for long periods

Symptoms from varicosities can range from cosmetic blemishes to mild to moderate pain. Discomfort is usually more pronounced at the end of the day or after a day spent standing or walking a lot. Occasionally, *superficial thrombophlebitis* (blood clots) in these veins can be a problem after pregnancy. These clots can be painful, but they are not dangerous; they don't travel to other parts of the body.

In severe cases, varicose veins may require treatment, including injection, ligation, stripping and laser treatment. It is rare to perform any of these procedures until you are finished childbearing.

Swelling and Water Retention

Swelling and water retention are a normal part of pregnancy; usually, you retain about 2.8 quarts (3 liters) of water. However, with extreme swelling, this amount can increase dramatically. Water retention occurs because of hormone changes and the blockage of blood flow by the enlarged uterus. It takes weeks for your uterus to return to its prepregnancy size, and consequently, it will be some time before you will get rid of this extra water.

To help lessen swelling, do the same things you were advised to do during pregnancy. It will help to lie on your side several times during the day and when you go to sleep. However, if you just sit in bed, it'll take longer to get rid of extra fluid; get up and get moving. Elevating your legs above the level of your heart is good, but lying on your side is better. Also, it is important to exercise regularly.

Headaches

Headaches can be a problem for some women after delivery. They do not usually indicate a problem, but they can certainly make you miserable.

Headaches may be caused or influenced by many factors—for example, a long labor, having to push for a while or if you have not slept in 24 to 36 hours. If you had pre-eclampsia (a variety of conditions including swelling, protein in urine or changes in reflexes) or pregnancy-induced hypertension (high blood pressure), these could both give you a headache.

An epidural or spinal anesthetic given during labor or for a C-section can result in a type of headache known as a *spinal headache*. This doesn't happen often—usually only once in every 100 deliveries—and is best treated with fluids and bed rest. Sometimes an epidural blood patch is used to seal the area of leakage from the spinal canal. With this procedure, the blood is withdrawn from your arm and introduced into the spinal canal. You are advised to lie flat on your back for 2 to 3 hours, so the blood can circulate in the spinal area and seal off any openings that may cause the headache.

Sometimes the stress of dealing with visitors and your new baby may contribute to your headaches. If you experience headaches, discuss the situation with your doctor. He or she can recommend a course of treatment for you. Usually rest, fluids and mild pain medicine offer relief.

It's important to tell your doctor if you have a headache that doesn't go away or get better, especially if a headache is severe or is accompanied by blurred vision or nausea.

Emotional Problems

You may experience many emotional changes after your baby is born. Mood swings, mild distress or bouts of crying are not uncommon. Changes in moods are often a result of the hormonal changes you experience after birth, just as they were when you were pregnant.

Sometimes the change in focus from you to the new baby can cause emotional upset. During your pregnancy, you were the center of attention; now the baby is. This abrupt change can make you feel very emotional. If you are prepared for this change, you may be less affected by it.

A lack of sleep may also play a part in how you feel. Many women are surprised by how tired they are emotionally *and* physically in the first few months after their baby's birth. Make sure you take time for yourself—you'll need a period of adjustment.

Sleep and rest can help you deal with mood shifts, which seem to occur more often when a woman is exhausted. Taking care of yourself is very important. See the discussion below and also see the discussion on the condition known as *postpartum distress* that begins on page 34.

Getting Enough Sleep and Rest

As many new parents—both fathers and mothers—can tell you, it's no easy task to adjust to night after night of interrupted sleep. A baby usually wakes up every 2 to 4 hours to feed. This can be disruptive to his parents, who probably wake up with him.

A cardinal rule with a newborn is "get sleep whenever and wherever you can." Until the baby is about 2 months old, you probably won't be able to put a long-term sleep plan into action. Other suggestions that might help include those below.

Involve Your Partner
Involve your partner in deciding who is going to do what at night. If you're breastfeeding, your partner can change the baby, then bring her to you every other night. After your milk becomes established, he could feed the baby a bottle of expressed milk. If you are bottlefeeding, he can feed the baby on alternate nights.

Be Sure the Baby Is Awake
Don't jump out of bed at your baby's first cry during the night. He may not really be awake yet and may not need tending. Give the baby a few minutes, and if he's still making noise, then go to him. You may be lucky and find that he goes back to sleep without you having to get up.

Turn in Earlier
You might not be able to rest during the day when the baby sleeps, but going to bed earlier may be more easily accomplished. Don't stay up late to watch the news or the late show. Go to bed around 8:30 or 9:00pm, if possible. This may mean you have to let some things go, but that's OK if it allows you to get some much-needed rest.

Get Daytime Help When Possible
The more support a couple has with their daily tasks and chores, the easier it will be to deal with sleepless nights. Ask friends and family to help. They probably won't be offended and may be glad you asked them for help.

Let things go when possible—the house doesn't have to be perfect, all the baby clothes and diapers don't have to be folded and put away, and the kitchen doesn't have to be spotless. Take it easy on yourself.

Changing Diapers
Make it as simple as possible to take care of your baby during the middle of the night. Be sure your baby's clothes are easy to work around. If a diaper isn't too wet, you may be able to let it go until the next feeding.

Exercise Every Day
Daily exercise can be great for you. Not strenuous exercise but any exercise that helps relieve some of the tension you may feel to help you sleep. A stroll around the block can be very beneficial. When possible, take your partner and baby with you to make it a family affair.

If You Have More Than One Baby

Recovery after the birth of twins, triplets or more may be a little more difficult for several reasons. Your pregnancy may have been harder on your body than a singleton pregnancy. The risk of problems or complications is higher with a multiple pregnancy. You may have gained more weight or experienced more swelling (edema). You may have had a Cesarean delivery. A multiple pregnancy usually delivers early, so you may not have had time to prepare to bring your babies home.

Gestation for a singleton pregnancy is about 280 days; for twins, about 260 days; and for triplets, about 247 days.

Another problem with early delivery is the possible prematurity of the babies. If your babies are premature and have to stay in the hospital, this can create emotional stress for you.

An added stress is that you will have two or more of everything—two or more diapers to change, babies to feed, clothes to wash and little bodies to bathe.

It's important to ask for help from family and friends. Don't be shy about this—many people are just waiting for you to ask. As you recover and the babies grow and get on some kind of schedule, life will go more smoothly.

No matter what, be sure you get enough rest. Your body needs time to recover, probably even more time than if you only had one baby. Be kind to yourself—you'll be glad you did.

Postpartum Distress

After your baby is born, you may be surprised by some of the emotions you feel. You have waited so long for this wonderful new life and have anticipated feelings of great joy and happiness. You may be surprised if you find yourself feeling feel sad and unhappy. You have delivered your baby, and the anticipation and excitement are over. You may wonder now if having a baby was a good idea. These feelings, called *postpartum distress*, are normal in many women (up to 80%).

In the past, postpartum distress was called "postpartum depression," and the entire range of feelings a woman might experience was lumped together under that term. Today, the general term is "postpartum distress," and we distinguish between the intensity of the feelings.

Many women experience some degree of postpartum distress. Most of the time, the feelings are mild; you may have heard them referred to as "baby blues" (see p. 35). These feelings usually appear between 2 days and 2 weeks after the baby is born. The situation is temporary and tends to leave as quickly as it comes. In unusual cases, it may last for several months and sometimes even more than a year.

Today, many experts consider some degree of postpartum distress normal. Some of the symptoms include:

- crying for no reason
- exhaustion
- irritability
- lack of confidence
- anxiety
- lack of feeling for the baby
- impatience
- low self-esteem
- oversensitivity
- restlessness

If you believe you are suffering from some of these symptoms, call your doctor. Almost all postpartum reactions are temporary and treatable.

Degrees of Postpartum Distress

The mildest form of postpartum distress is *baby blues*. This situation lasts only a couple of weeks, and symptoms do not worsen. See the description above.

A more-serious form of postpartum distress is called *postpartum depression* (PPD); it affects about 10 percent of all new mothers. The difference between baby blues and postpartum depression is in the frequency, intensity and duration of symptoms. Having problems sleeping is one way to distinguish between the two. If you can sleep while someone else tends the baby, it is probably baby blues. If you can't sleep because of anxiety, it may be PPD.

PPD can occur any time from 2 weeks to 1 year after birth. A mother may have feelings of anger, confusion, panic and hopelessness. Her eating and sleeping patterns may change. She may be fearful that she will hurt her baby or is not taking good care of her baby. She may think she is a bad mother or feel as if she is going crazy. Anxiety is a major symptom of PPD.

The most-serious form of postpartum distress is called *postpartum psychosis*. In this situation, the woman may have hallucinations, think about suicide or try to harm the baby.

What Causes Postpartum Distress?

We don't know exactly what causes postpartum distress; not every woman experiences it. We believe hormonal changes are part of it.

Many demands are placed on a new mother, which can cause distress. Other possible factors being considered include a family history of depression, little support after the birth, isolation and fatigue.

Ways to Deal with the Problem

One way to deal with the problem is to have a good cry, if you feel like one. Some researchers believe that emotional tears play a part in helping the body deal with stress—it may also evoke sympathy in those around you. Because baby blues may be related to stress, a good cry may be beneficial for you.

You can help yourself in other ways, too. Begin before the baby's birth. Set up a support network; ask family members and friends to help. Have your mother or mother-in-law stay with you to help out for a while. Maybe your partner can take some leave. Consider hiring someone to come in and help each day.

There is no treatment for baby blues other than emotional support, but there are ways you can help ease symptoms. In addition to asking for help, rest whenever the baby sleeps. Talk to your partner; it may be hard for him to help if he doesn't know you're having a hard time. Finding other mothers who are in the same situation will enable you to share your feelings and experiences. There may be some support groups in your area—ask your doctor for the names of groups. Keep the number of visitors to a small group. Entertaining guests can be exhausting and very stressful for you. Don't be too hard on yourself—let some things slide. Take care of yourself. Exercise every day. Eat healthfully, drink plenty of fluids and avoid alcohol. Try to get out of the house at least once every day.

With postpartum depression, the situation is a little more serious. Use the above suggestions. In addition, medication may be necessary to help relieve some symptoms. Research indicates about 85% of all women who suffer from postpartum depression require medication, including antidepressants, tranquilizers and hormones; often they are used together. No single treatment has been shown to be more effective than another.

If you breastfeed, medication selection may be more limited. Certain medications, such as Pamelor®, Prozac® and Norpramin®, can be used by a woman while breastfeeding. The baby's doctor must be aware of it, and the baby must be monitored for side effects. Discuss the situation with your OB/GYN and your pediatrician if medication is prescribed to you while you are breastfeeding.

Postpartum Distress Can Affect Your Partner
If you experience baby blues or PPD, it can affect your partner. Prepare your partner for this situation before your baby is born. Explain to him that if it happens to you, it's only temporary.

There are some things you might suggest to your partner to do for himself if you get blue or depressed.

- Tell him not to take the situation personally.
- Suggest he talk to friends, family members, other fathers or a professional.
- He should eat well, get enough rest and exercise.
- Ask him to be patient with you.
- Ask him to support you. He can provide you with his love and support during this difficult time.

Will We Ever Have Sex Again?

Probably the last thing on your mind right now is resuming sexual relations. Many women express the feeling that sex at this time is too much to cope with. They need to rest, get enough sleep and get back into a routine before they start thinking about sex again.

Resuming sexual relations can be a little difficult. You are naturally concerned about pain. The best thing you can do for yourself is to take it easy and go slowly. Don't have sexual intercourse until you feel ready. Involve your partner by sharing your feelings and concerns.

Your sex drive, and that of your partner, can be affected by stress, emotions and fatigue. There are also actual physical reasons why you may not feel like having sex. These include your changing estrogen levels, which can cause vaginal dryness and irritation. You are probably still bleeding, too. If you had an episiotomy, that may add to your discomfort. And with all the changes your body has gone through, you just may not feel sexy right now. That's OK.

In the past, we advised a woman to wait at least 6 weeks before having intercourse. Today we tell a woman to let her body be her guide, but 6 weeks is still a good suggestion. You probably won't feel like it anyway until then. If you feel no pain or discomfort, and your episiotomy is healed, you can resume sexual relations as soon as you feel up to it. Just be sure the bleeding has stopped. For most women, this is at least 4 to 6 weeks after delivery. Talk to your partner to make sure he isn't expecting to resume relations with you 1 or 2 weeks after delivery, when you're thinking it will be 4 to 6 weeks!

When you do decide to have sex again, you can take some steps to make the experience more enjoyable for both of you. Try the following.

Steps for Resuming Sexual Relations

- Be sure you are healed enough to have sexual intercourse.
- Use lots of lubricant to relieve vaginal dryness and to avoid irritation from friction (but avoid petroleum jelly if you use condoms).
- If you use the woman-on-top position, you can control the amount of penetration.
- Try experimenting with foreplay to add life to your sexual experience.
- Don't focus on your body and the way it looks; if your partner says you're attractive, believe him.
- Remember, there are alternatives to sexual intercourse. Simply kissing and caressing can be great turn-ons.

If you do decide to have intercourse, you need to take precautions if you don't want to get pregnant again immediately; you can become pregnant before you have a menstrual period. Read the section on birth control that follows.

Birth Control after Pregnancy

Contraception after the birth of your baby is important and is something you probably need to think about. Most women begin ovulating 6 to 8 weeks after birth if they are not breastfeeding—if you have unprotected sex when you ovulate, you could get pregnant again. Breastfeeding can delay ovulation and menstrual periods for a few months. If you don't want to have another baby very soon, it's important to discuss birth-control options with your partner and your doctor in the hospital or at your 6-week postpartum checkup.

We know that breastfeeding protects you against pregnancy to some degree, but breastfeeding is *not* an effective method of birth control by itself! If you breastfeed, it's important to consider birth-control methods if you don't want to get pregnant.

If you used a diaphragm or cervical cap for birth control before pregnancy, you will need to be refitted after delivery. The size of the cervix or vagina often changes after a woman has a baby. Condoms and spermicides are OK to use if you breastfeed.

Oral contraceptives (birth-control pills) are also available. They are easy to use and pose few health risks, so many women choose this method of contraception. In the past, oral contraceptives were not prescribed for a breastfeeding woman. However, today we have progestin-only pills available, often called *minipills*. They do not decrease milk production, and there are no known harmful effects on the baby. Most doctors do not prescribe these oral contraceptives until a woman's milk supply is fully established, usually 1 to 2 weeks after birth or by the time of your 6-week postpartum checkup. If you are bottlefeeding and want to use a birth-control pill that contains estrogen and progestin (the regular birth-control pill), wait at least 2 weeks after delivery to begin.

An IUD is the method of choice for some women. Depending on the type of IUD, it can remain there for up to 8 years once inserted, with very few problems. An IUD has no effect on milk production, so it may also be used after a baby's birth. You must wait until 6 weeks after delivery to have an IUD put in place.

You may decide on a method that can be started immediately after delivery. Norplant® is a small rod containing progesterone that is placed under the skin of your arm to provide birth control for an extended period. Depo-Provera® is a hormone injection given every 3 months. Both methods are acceptable for bottlefeeding and breastfeeding moms.

Putting It All in Perspective

The concerns we've discussed in this chapter are ones many women face each day. It's important to know that most of them are temporary and won't interfere greatly with life with your new baby.

The key to dealing with anything during your recovery period is to relax. Any of these situations is more easily dealt with if you don't become stressed by it.

CHAPTER 4

Feeding Your Baby

Feeding your baby is one of the most important things you can do for her. The nutrition your child receives from you while you're pregnant and from birth gives her the start in life she needs to grow and to develop through childhood into adulthood. Now that you have given birth, it is important for both you and your baby to continue to eat healthily.

You probably have many questions about what is right for you and your baby. Read this section dealing with breastfeeding and bottle-feeding, and talk to other mothers to get their advice. The more information you have, the better able you will be to make decisions about this most-important aspect of caring for your baby.

Feeding a Newborn

When a baby is hungry, he exhibits definite signs, such as fussing, putting his hands in his mouth, and turning his head and opening his mouth when his cheek is touched.

Most newborns feed every 3 to 4 hours, although some feed as often as every 2 hours. You may decide to feed your baby at regular intervals to help him get on a schedule, or you may decide to let your baby set his own schedule—some babies need to nurse more often than others do. Sometimes a baby needs to feed more often than usual, especially during periods of growth.

The baby himself is normally the best judge of how much he needs at each feeding. Usually, a baby will turn away from the nipple (mother or bottle) when he is full.

Some people may suggest that you feed your baby water instead of breast milk or formula. Whether this is a good idea for your baby depends on many things, including your baby's weight, how well she is doing and whether she is hungry or thirsty. Your healthcare provider will advise you.

If you are able to breastfeed, it is usually the best way to feed your baby. Breast milk is easily digested and contains every nutrient your baby needs. Research has found that breastfed babies have lower rates of infection because of the immunological content of breast milk. Breastfeeding provides the baby with a sense of security and gives the mother a sense of self-esteem. However, if there are reasons you cannot or choose not to breastfeed, be assured that your baby will also do well on formula.

It won't harm your baby if you cannot or choose not to breastfeed. No mother should feel guilty if she doesn't wish to breastfeed her baby. Sometimes breastfeeding is not possible because of a physical condition or other problem; a woman may also choose not to breastfeed because of other demands on her time, such as a job or other children to care for. An infant can still get all the love, attention and nutrition she needs if breastfeeding is not possible.

If You Choose to Bottlefeed

Although some women may feel that they are not good mothers if they choose not to breastfeed, they are not alone—statistics show that more women choose to bottlefeed than breastfeed their babies. Your baby can receive good nutrition if you bottlefeed with iron-fortified formula, so don't feel guilty if you opt to bottlefeed.

Bottlefeeding offers many advantages that are often overlooked. Some women enjoy the freedom bottlefeeding provides. It enables others in the family, such as the father, to help care for the baby; many fathers appreciate being more involved in caring for their child. Bottlefed babies are often able to go longer between feedings because formula is usually digested more slowly than breast milk. Bottlefeeding also helps you to determine exactly how much your baby is taking in at each feeding. Bottlefed babies take from 2 to 3 ounces of formula at a feeding, and usually feed every 3 to 4 hours for the first month.

You may have twins or triplets (or even more); these babies are often bottlefed because it is more difficult and demanding to breast-feed multiple babies. Some women pump their breast milk and divide it between the babies, then supplement the breast milk with formula. Other mothers use only formula to feed multiples. Still others try to breastfeed one or two babies at each nursing, giving any other babies formula for that feeding. It's important to know that if you have more than one baby, there are many ways you can provide your babies with the nutrition they need.

When you bottlefeed, there are some tips to keep in mind to help make the experience a healthy and happy one for you and your baby.

Tips for Bottlefeeding

- Wash your hands before you prepare formula.
- Clean all feeding equipment thoroughly before use.
- Check formula expiration dates to ensure the formula has not expired.
- If you prepare formula or bottles ahead of time, keep them refrigerated.
- Throw away all leftover formula.
- Get rid of bottle nipples that are hard or stiff.

Some parents fear that bottlefeeding will not encourage bonding between them and their child. However, there are ways you can bottlefeed your baby that will help develop a closer bond between you. Try the following ideas.

- Snuggle your baby close to you during feeding.
- Heat formula to body temperature by running the filled bottle under warm water. There's no evidence that feeding refrigerated formula without warming it will harm your baby.
- Remove the bottle during feeding to allow your baby to rest. It usually takes 10 minutes or longer to finish feeding.

Safety Precautions

- Don't leave the baby alone with the bottle. Never prop up a bottle and leave the baby alone to suck on it as he may choke on the bottle, he may not get burped, and there's evidence that he may suffer from tooth decay when his teeth do come in. Remember that feeding times are important for bonding with your baby.
- Never put a baby down to bed with a bottle.

Types of Formula to Use When Bottlefeeding
There are many different types of formula you can choose to feed your baby. Most babies do very well on milk-based formula, but some need specialized formulas. Several types are available on the market today, including:

- milk-based, lactose-free formula for babies with feeding problems, such as fussiness, gas, vomiting and diarrhea caused by lactose intolerance
- soy-based, lactose-free formula for babies with cow's-milk allergies or sensitivity to cow's milk
- hypoallergenic protein formula, which is lactose-free and easier to digest for babies with colic or other symptoms of milk-protein allergy

Research has shown that feeding a baby with a bottle that is slanted is better. This design keeps the nipple full of milk, which means the baby takes in less air. Swallowing air can be a cause of discomfort to your baby. A slanted bottle also helps ensure the baby is sitting up to drink. When a baby drinks lying down, milk can pool in the Eustachian tube, and this can cause ear infections.

The American Academy of Pediatrics recommends that a baby be fed iron-fortified formula for the first year of life. Feeding iron-fortified formula for a year helps to maintain adequate iron intake.

If You Choose to Breastfeed

Many women choose to breastfeed their babies. It's a healthy way to feed your baby, and it helps to create a close bond between the mother and child.

You can usually begin breastfeeding your baby within an hour after birth, which provides your baby with *colostrum*, the first milk your breasts produce. Colostrum helps boost the baby's immune system. Breastfeeding also causes your pituitary gland to release *oxytocin*, the hormone that causes your uterus to contract and keeps bleeding to a minimum.

Don't be discouraged if you experience difficulty when you first start breastfeeding. It takes some time to find out what works for you and your baby. Hold your baby in such a way that she can reach your breast easily while nursing, either across your chest or lying down in bed. Your baby should take your nipple fully into her mouth, so that her gums cover the *areola*, the pigmented area around the nipple. She can't suck effectively if your nipple is only slightly drawn into her mouth.

If you have more than one baby, you should be able to breastfeed them all. You may find it a little more challenging, but many mothers have done it. You may have to try a creative approach, but with time, you'll probably work it out satisfactorily. For example, you may choose to pump your breasts and divide the breast milk between (or among) your babies, then supplement with formula. Or you may breastfeed your babies for a short while every time they nurse, then alternate feeding them formula. Or you may try to breastfeed exclusively. Studies have shown that frequent nursing stimulates milk production. Talk with your physician and your pediatrician about what might work best for you.

Breastfeeding is an excellent way to bond with your baby because of the physical closeness established during the feeding process. However, there are also other ways you can bond with your baby. Studies show that carrying your baby close to your body in a slinglike carrier on your chest or back helps the bonding process. This is also a great way for dads to bond with their baby.

An added benefit to breastfeeding that is becoming more widely known is the presence of DHA in breast milk. DHA (decosahexanoic acid) is the primary structural fatty acid that makes up the retina of the eye and the gray matter of the brain. During pregnancy, your baby receives this important substance through the placenta. After birth, your breast milk continues to supply your baby with DHA. Why is this important for your baby? Studies have shown that a baby with DHA in his diet may have a higher IQ and greater visual development than babies fed formula without DHA.

It's nearly impossible for a baby to become allergic to its mother's breast milk; breastfeeding may in fact prevent milk allergies. This is important if there is a history of allergies in your family or your partner's family. The longer a baby breastfeeds, the less likely he is to be exposed to substances that could cause allergy problems.

Recent studies have found additional valid reasons for a mother to nurse her baby. We now know that breast milk contains more benefits than you can imagine. Listed below are some of the important reasons to breastfeed.

Important Reasons to Breastfeed Your Baby

- Breast milk offers protection from infection. The incidence of ear infections is significantly reduced in infants who breastfeed for longer than 4 months. It may help prevent diarrhea in infants and may also inhibit the growth of bacteria that cause urinary-tract infections (UTIs).
- The baby's permanent teeth may come in straighter.
- The risk of breast cancer may be quite a bit lower for women who were breastfed.
- Breastfeeding may lower the risk of a baby developing juvenile diabetes, lymphoma and Crohn's disease later in life.
- Women who breastfeed may have an easier time losing weight after delivery, as their metabolism may be speeded up a little.

Disadvantages to Breastfeeding
The greatest disadvantage for many mothers who choose to breastfeed is that this ties them down so completely to the baby. Because a mother must be available when her baby is hungry, breastfeeding can sometimes make other family members feel left out.

A mother who breastfeeds must pay careful attention to her diet, both for the nourishment she takes in and the avoidance of foods and substances that may pass into her breast milk and cause problems for the baby. Most substances you eat or drink (or take orally, such as medications) can pass through your breast milk to your baby. Spicy foods, chocolate and caffeine are just a few things your baby can react to when you ingest them. Be careful about what you eat and drink while breastfeeding. Caffeine in breast milk can cause irritability and sleeplessness in a breastfed baby.

Tips for Breastfeeding Mothers

It's not always easy to get started breastfeeding, even though you probably think it's the most natural thing in the world to do. (It is, but it still takes practice!) Below are some tips to keep in mind.

- Relax in a comfortable place before you start. Make this a peaceful experience.
- Make sure your baby is comfortable, too. Be sure he's dry and warm.
- Help your baby connect with your breast by brushing your nipple across the baby's lips. When she opens her mouth, place the nipple and as much of the areola in her mouth as you can. You should feel her pull the breast while sucking, without this being painful. If you experience pain, disengage her by slipping your finger into the corner of her mouth and gently pulling down to break the suction.
- Don't rush—it takes longer for baby to nurse than to drink a bottle; it may take up to 20 or 25 minutes.

Warning Signs during Breastfeeding

You need to take extra-special care of yourself when you breastfeed. Below are some signs that might indicate you are having a problem. If you experience *any* of these problems, call your doctor immediately:

- fever or chills
- extreme fatigue and body aches, as if you have the flu
- burning pain in either or both breasts
- red streaks on the breast
- lumpy areas in your breasts
- a feeling of warmth in either breast
- swollen breasts, which keep the baby from latching on to the nipple
- sore, cracked or bleeding nipples
- milk that does not flow freely
- low milk supply
- any feelings of depression or extreme sadness

Warning Signs to Watch for in Your Baby

Warning signs may also be noticed in your baby. If you experience any of the following with your infant, call your pediatrician.

- The baby doesn't wake up or stay awake long enough to nurse.

- The baby is fussy after nursing, and cannot be settled by feeding again.
- The baby has fewer than two bowel movements a day.
- The baby has signs of jaundice.

Your Milk Production

Some women worry that they will not have enough breast milk to feed their baby. This is not a common problem, even for mothers of twins or triplets. With some practice and lots of patience, nearly every woman can breastfeed her baby (or babies).

If you want to have breast milk available so your baby can drink it while you are away from him, you can "express" it. Do this by using a breast pump (hand, battery or electrically operated) to remove milk from your breasts. Expressed milk can be refrigerated or frozen, and saved for later use. Breast milk doesn't need immediate refrigeration; it will stay fresh for up to 4 hours at temperatures as high as 77°F (25°C) and 24 hours at 60°F (15.5°C).

It takes some time to express your milk. You'll need 10 to 30 minutes to do it, depending on the type of pump you have. Electric pumps work the best; they can be rented at many medical supply stores. You'll probably have to do it one to four times a day (around the time you would normally nurse). You need a comfortable, private place where you can relax enough for the milk to flow into your breasts—this is known as *milk letdown*. (See pages 49 and 52 for an explanation of milk letdown.)

Storing and Freezing Breast Milk

Store your breast milk after you express it. There are several steps you can take to store breast milk safely.

- Pump or express your breast milk into a clean container.
- Label the container with the date and amount of breast milk collected.
- You can keep fresh breast milk at room temperature for a few hours; it's best to refrigerate it as soon as possible.
- Breast milk can be safely stored in the refrigerator for up to 72 hours.

You can even freeze breast milk. It can be kept in a refrigerator freezer for 6 months or in a deep freezer (–20°F; –29°C) for up to 12 months. Fill the container only 3/4 full, to allow for expansion during freezing. Freeze breast milk in small portions, such as 2 to 4 ounces (56 to 112g), because these amounts thaw more quickly. *Don't* thaw breast milk in the microwave—radiation can destroy substances in the milk that help protect an infant from infection.

You can combine fresh breast milk with frozen breast milk. First, cool the fresh, newly expressed breast milk before combining it with the frozen breast milk. The amount of thawed breast milk must be more than the amount of fresh breast milk. Never refreeze breast milk! Below are ways to thaw breast milk so that you can ensure it maintains its high quality.

- Put the container of frozen milk in a bowl of warm water for 30 minutes, or hold the frozen container under warm running water.
- Never microwave breast milk; the radiation can alter its composition and destroy substances that protect your baby from infection.
- Swirl the container to blend any fat that might have separated during thawing.
- Feed the thawed milk to your baby immediately, or store it in the refrigerator for up to 24 hours.

It's best to avoid alternately bottlefeeding your baby with formula, if you have a choice. Your milk supply is driven by your baby's demand. Breastfed babies eat about every 2 to 3 hours in the first few weeks of life. If you bottlefeed formula part of the time, your baby won't demand the breast milk from you, and your body will slow down its production.

Some Common Problems during Breastfeeding

Breast milk becomes more plentiful between 2 days and 6 days after birth, when it changes from colostrum to mature milk. Your breasts may become engorged, and you may have some pain for 24 to 36 hours. Continue breastfeeding during this time, even if your breasts are sore. Wear a bra that offers good support, and apply cold compresses to your breasts for short periods to ease the soreness. Take acetaminophen (Tylenol®) if pain is severe, but don't take anything stronger unless your physician prescribes it.

Soon after your baby begins to nurse, you will experience the tingling or cramping in your breasts known as milk letdown. This means milk is flowing into the breast ducts and usually occurs several times during feeding. Occasionally, a baby will choke a bit when the milk comes too quickly.

Sore Nipples

Your nipples may become sore when you begin breastfeeding. If your baby doesn't take your nipple into her mouth fully during breastfeeding, her jaws can compress the nipple, which makes it sore. However, it's good to know that sore nipples rarely last longer than a couple of days. Continue breastfeeding, even if your nipples are sore.

There are other ways to help avoid sore nipples. Nipple shields can be worn inside your bra between the nipple and bra fabric to provide some relief. They prevent your tender skin from rubbing on the bra fabric. A mild cream can also be applied to soothe sore nipples. Ask your pharmacist or healthcare provider to recommend products that are OK to use during nursing.

Breast Infections

Be aware that you can get a breast infection while you are breastfeeding. Large red streaks that extend up the breast toward the armpit usually indicate a breast infection. Call your healthcare provider immediately because an infection can cause a fever to develop within 4 to 8 hours after the appearance of the red streaks. Antibiotic treatment should be started immediately. Medical treatment can improve the symptoms, and the infection may even clear up within 24 hours.

Apply a warm compress to the affected area, or soak the breast in warm water. Express milk or breastfeed while massaging the tender area.

If you develop flulike symptoms with a sore breast, call your doctor. Antibiotic treatment may need to be started. You may need to rest in bed, but first empty your infected breast by pumping or breastfeeding every hour or two. If a breast infection is left untreated, it can turn into an abscess. This is very painful and may need to be opened and drained.

There are several things you can do to help prevent a breast infection. Eat right, and get plenty of rest. This can help reduce stress and keep your immune system working efficiently. Don't wear tight-fitting bras, especially underwire types because these can block your normal milk flow, which may cause an infection. Empty your breasts on a regular schedule to avoid engorgement. After each feeding or pumping, let your nipples air-dry for a few minutes.

Don't stop nursing if you get a breast infection—if you stop nursing, the infection may get worse. This occurs because you are still making milk, and stopping breastfeeding will make your breasts even more engorged and painful.

Plugged Milk Ducts

Another situation you might encounter during breastfeeding is a *plugged milk duct*. A plugged milk duct prevents breast milk from flowing freely. It results in tender or firm areas of the breast becoming more painful after breastfeeding. A plugged duct is not red, and you will not have a fever.

Treatment is usually unnecessary with a plugged duct. It usually takes care of itself if you continue to nurse frequently. Applying warm compresses to the sore area helps with the pain, and may help open the duct. Acetaminophen (Tylenol®) may be used for pain.

Colds and Viruses

If you have a cold or other virus, it's all right to breastfeed. If you're taking an antibiotic, it's OK to breastfeed as long as you know the drug is not incompatible with nursing. Ask your doctor or pharmacist if any medication prescribed for you should not be taken while breastfeeding. Be sure to ask *before* you begin taking it.

Other Common Breastfeeding Concerns

Nursing in Public

Some women feel uncomfortable breastfeeding their baby in public. In many countries, breastfeeding in public is a natural part of life. If you feel uncomfortable nursing in a public place, go into the ladies' room or a secluded lounge, and feed your baby there. Look at each instance by itself—you'll soon learn how comfortable you feel feeding your baby away from home.

Your Baby's Nursing Pattern

You may be unprepared for how often your baby will want (and need) to nurse in the first week after birth. You may wonder if it's worth it to continue. Relax and be patient—it takes time for your baby to develop his nursing pattern. By the end of the second or third week, a pattern will probably become established, and your baby will sleep longer between feedings.

Burping Your Baby
It's a good idea to burp your baby regularly after each feeding; some babies even need to be burped during a feeding. There are various ways to burp your baby, such as holding him over your shoulder or sitting him in your lap and gently rubbing or patting his back. You may want to place a towel over your shoulder or at least have one handy in case he spits up. If your baby doesn't burp, don't try to force it.

When Your Baby Vomits
Babies frequently spit up some breast milk or formula after a feeding. This is common in the early months because the muscle at the top of her stomach has not fully developed. When a baby spits up enough to propel the stomach contents several inches, it is called *projectile vomiting*. If your baby vomits after a feeding, don't feed her again immediately, as her stomach may be upset. It may be wise to wait until the next feeding.

Medications
Be careful with medications. Although there are many situations in which medication is beneficial for you, in some instances it can have a negative effect on your baby. Take a medication *only* when you really need it. Ask your physician for the smallest dose possible. Check with your OB-GYN and your pediatrician to see if it's OK to use the medication while breastfeeding. Ask about any potential effects on the baby, so you'll be alert for them. Postpone treatment, if possible.

If you take a medication immediately after nursing, it may have less of an effect on the baby. If a medication would have a serious effect on your baby, you may decide to bottlefeed her for the time that you must take the medication. You can maintain your milk supply by pumping (then throwing away) your expressed milk.

Reasons to Avoid Bottles
If possible, it's best to avoid bottles for the first month of breastfeeding for two reasons: your baby may come to prefer feeding from a bottle (it's not as hard to suck), and your breasts may not produce enough milk.

How Long to Breastfeed
Nursing during the first 4 weeks of your baby's life provides the most effective form of protection for your baby and the most-beneficial hormone release to help you recover after the birth. Nursing for the first

6 months is also very beneficial for your baby; it provides excellent nutrition and protection from illness. After 6 months, the nutrition and protection aspects are not as critical for your baby. If you can nurse for only a short period of time, try to stick with it for the first 6 months or at least for the first 4 weeks.

Breastfeeding While at Work or Away
You can continue breastfeeding your baby after you return to work, although if you breastfeed exclusively, you will have to pump your breasts or arrange to see your baby during the day. Alternatively, you can nurse your baby at home, and substitute formula when you're at work.

You may find it necessary to be away from your baby for a few days during breastfeeding. If this is so, you will probably need to pump your breast milk while you are gone. If you don't, you may be very uncomfortable because the breast milk will continue to flow in. Take a breast pump with you and discard the breast milk after it is pumped.

What to Wear When Breastfeeding
It may be more comfortable to wear a nursing bra if you breastfeed. These have cups that open so you can breastfeed without having to get undressed. They also provide very good support for your enlarged breasts.

There are other special clothes you might want to consider wearing if you are breastfeeding. Nightgowns, shift dresses and full-cut blouses have been designed with discreet breast openings so you don't have to get undressed to breastfeed. You can reach up inside your outer clothing, unhook your nursing bra and place your baby at your breast without anyone noticing. Lightly draping a towel or baby blanket over your shoulder and over the baby's head adds further coverage.

The Milk-Letdown Response
Be aware that your nipples will drip milk when your baby, or any other baby you are around, cries. This is called the *milk-letdown response*. Many mothers don't understand that this is normal and become very upset when it occurs the first time. To protect your clothing, be sure you wear breast shields or breast pads inside your bra.

Breastfeeding With Chronic Illness
Some breastfeeding mothers have special problems they must deal with. If you have a chronic illness, you may need to make certain changes in your diet, medication use or daily activities. Discuss these with your doctor.

Breastfeeding after Breast Surgery
Many women who have had breast-enlargement surgery are able to breastfeed successfully. Even if you have had breast-reduction surgery, you should still be able to breastfeed without any problems. The surgery may result in decreased milk production, but usually your breasts will still produce enough milk to nurse your baby.

Switching Breasts during Breastfeeding
It's a good idea to switch breasts regularly during breastfeeding, but wait until your baby finishes with one breast before switching to the other one. The consistency of breast milk changes from thinner to richer as the baby nurses. At the next feeding, start your baby on the breast you nursed last. This helps you keep both breasts stimulated. If your baby only wants to nurse from one breast each feeding, simply switch to the other breast the next feeding.

Problems While Breastfeeding
If you experience problems while breastfeeding, many hospitals have breastfeeding specialists you can call on for help. Personnel at your doctor's office may be able to refer you to someone knowledgeable. You can also look in the telephone book for the La Leche League, an organization that promotes breastfeeding. Someone from your local chapter will be able to give you advice and encouragement.

Stopping Nursing

When you decide to discontinue nursing, you can either taper off gradually or stop cold turkey. Each way has its advantages. If you want to taper off gradually, start a bottle every other feeding, or offer bottles during the day and nurse at night. In the past, medications were given to stop milk production, but because of safety concerns, these are no longer used. If you stop "cold turkey," you may experience some sleepless nights from a screaming baby, and you may have physical discomfort from engorged breasts. However, this method takes less time.

Some women like to nurse until they return to work. Others nurse through the first year. It all depends on your personal situation and preference, and when your baby starts to get his teeth!

CHAPTER 5

Nutrition to Get Back in Shape

After a woman gives birth, one of her first concerns is usually regaining her prepregnancy figure. Some women mistakenly believe they can get in shape and look better faster if they go on a "crash" diet, cutting calories to lose the weight they gained during pregnancy. While this may seem like a good idea, it really isn't. Your body needs time to recover from the grueling 9-month experience that has just ended. If you are nursing, hormone adjustments are taking place. In addition, when you undergo a crash diet, your body can release environmental toxins, like pesticides, that are stored in your body fat. These can get into your bloodstream and may contaminate your breast milk.

Nearly every woman gains some extra weight during pregnancy to help her deal with the postpartum demands on her body. Even if you don't breastfeed, your body adds extra fat to prepare for this important event. Nature also knows that a new mother needs extra energy, and the fat the body lays down during pregnancy prepares for this need. Cutting your calories isn't going to help your body meet the many demands on it; therefore, a nutritious eating plan is the best course of action.

Following the birth of your baby, you probably lost between 10 and 20 pounds (4.5 to 9kg). You may have been expecting to lose more, but there are some practical reasons why you did not. Your body retains quite a lot of fluid, especially if you have an I.V. Your breasts will also be *engorged*, or filled with fluid. Both of these conditions add to your overall body weight. However, in the days following the birth, your body will flush out the extra fluid and will begin to regulate its milk production. When this happens, you'll see your weight begin to drop.

It takes time to get your figure back; the best way to accomplish this task is to eat nutritiously, develop and follow an exercise program, and realize that it's going to take time! Below is a discussion of some of the nutrition tips that have worked for women all over the world in helping them to regain their prepregnancy figures.

Getting Back in Shape

When you're getting back in shape, it's important to follow a nutritious eating plan, such as the one you followed during pregnancy. Rest assured, however, that if your diet is less than perfect (and whose *is* perfect anyway?), your body will endeavor to make breast milk that contains all the essential nutrients necessary for your baby's good health.

You need to continue to eat foods high in complex carbohydrates, such as grain products, fruits and vegetables. Lean meats, chicken and fish are good sources of protein. For your dairy products, choose the low-fat or skim-milk types.

A good plan to follow for each day is to eat a variety of foods that contain all the nutrients your body needs. Try to eat these foods in a form as close to their natural state as possible. You don't have to eat three big meals a day; you may prefer to eat the necessary calories spread out over five or six small meals. Eating many small meals helps to keep your energy levels stable. Another suggestion is to eat a combination of protein, carbohydrates and a little bit of fat each time you eat. This takes longer to digest and helps keep your blood-sugar level up.

If you are bottlefeeding, you need fewer calories than you would if you were breastfeeding. However, don't cut your caloric intake drastically in the hopes of losing weight quickly. You still need to eat nutritiously to maintain good energy levels. Whatever you do, make sure the calories you are eating do not come from junk foods.

We've included information on the types and quantities of foods to eat per day, both for breastfeeding mothers and mothers who choose to bottlefeed. (See pp. 59–61.) Choose nine servings from the bread/ cereal/pasta and rice group if you breastfeed and six servings if you bottlefeed. Servings of fruit should be four for breastfeeding women and three for mothers who bottlefeed. Eat five servings of vegetables if you nurse and three servings if you don't. Eat three servings from the dairy group while breastfeeding and two servings if you bottlefeed. The amount of protein in your diet should be 8 ounces if breastfeeding and 6 ounces if bottlefeeding. Be particularly careful with fats, oils and sugars; limit your intake to 4 teaspoons if nursing and 3 teaspoons if not.

During breastfeeding, you need to continue to keep your fluid intake high, just as you did during pregnancy. In order for your body to produce 20 to 30 ounces of milk each day, your fluid intake is crucial. If you don't drink extra fluids, you could become dehydrated, as your body attempts to get the fluid somewhere. Plan to drink a glass of water every time you sit down to nurse your baby. Drink plenty of water or other beverages to help you meet this goal, but avoid beverages that are high in calories, such as sodas, or caffeinated or alcoholic beverages, which tend to dehydrate the body (see p. 58).

Nutrition Plan for Breastfeeding

Breastfeeding can be good for you, as well as for your baby. Studies have shown that a woman who breastfeeds may lose weight more quickly after the birth of her baby than a woman who bottlefeeds and eats fewer calories. Making breast milk is a strenuous job, and your body may respond by burning more calories, which will help you lose weight faster. Other studies demonstrate that some women do not lose weight quickly, which can also be influenced by their metabolism. As during pregnancy, you may be eating for two, but you don't have to eat twice as much!

Vitamin and Mineral Supplements
A well-balanced diet during breastfeeding helps you maintain energy levels and better physical health. Your doctor may recommend that you continue taking your *prenatal vitamins* if you plan to breastfeed. (Prenatal vitamins are multivitamins that contain extra iron and folic acid.) Your body can use the extra nutrients during this important time. Some women take them throughout their baby's first year.

You may also need supplemental iron, especially if you lost a lot of blood at delivery. Ask your doctor about this before you leave the hospital. Even if you don't need extra iron, it's a good idea to eat foods rich in this mineral to ensure your continued good health. Iron-rich foods include meats; liver; dark-green leafy vegetables, such as spinach, kale and chard; dried beans; dried fruits and whole-grain products.

Other vitamins and minerals you need include calcium, zinc, magnesium, folic acid, vitamin B_6 and vitamin D. Calcium is necessary for bone strength—yours! You can get calcium from dairy products (you can choose low-fat products, if you prefer) and some calcium-fortified food products, such as orange juice. Zinc, important for wound healing and the health of your immune system, can be found in seafoods, such as clams, mussels and crabmeat; it is also found in beef and the dark meat of chicken or turkey. Magnesium is essential for healthy muscles and bones; good sources include bran cereal, spinach, lentils, white potatoes and winter squash. Folic acid, now added to many foods in the United States, is necessary for healthy blood cells. Lentils, spinach, broccoli, orange juice and various beans are excellent sources. Vitamin B_6 helps your body metabolize foods and helps to maintain your central-nervous-system (CNS) function. Chicken, fish, some beans and pork are good sources. Vitamin D is a must for proper calcium absorption. Milk is the best source, but be careful—too much vitamin D can be toxic!

Are There Foods to Avoid If I'm Breastfeeding?

You've probably heard that some foods you consume may cause problems for your baby. This is true. It's also true that other substances you ingest, such as some medications, can also cause problems for your nursing infant. It's a good idea to think along the lines that "anything I eat may pass into my breast milk, and thus to my nursing baby." If you're unsure whether you should eat something, or if it is OK to take a particular substance, especially medicine of some kind, ask your doctor *before* you take it.

Many women ask about caffeine and alcohol. We know that both of these substances can pass into your breast milk, so use caution when you eat foods or drink beverages that contain them.

Caffeine

Caffeine passes into your breast milk but only in small amounts. If you take in moderate amounts, such as drinking three or four cups of coffee a day, it probably won't affect your baby. However, if you notice any fussiness or wakefulness in your baby, gradually cut back on your caffeine intake to see if it makes a difference. It is probably best to keep your caffeine intake to no more than four cups a day.

Alcohol Intake

Yes, you may have an alcoholic beverage while breastfeeding, as long as you take a drink only occasionally, and limit your intake. We know that alcohol passes into breast milk very quickly; it also passes out very quickly. If you drink a glass of beer or wine, it will pass out of your breast milk within about 3 hours after consumption. So if you're going to drink alcohol, consume it immediately after breastfeeding so that your body has time to metabolize it before your baby nurses again.

Too much alcohol can affect both your baby and your milk production. It can make your baby very lethargic and can inhibit milk production in you.

Cigarettes and Tobacco

Avoid smoking and smoky atmospheres whenever possible. Not only is smoking bad for your own health, but it can be detrimental to the health of your baby. Secondary smoking has been shown to be a contributing cause in cases of sudden-infant-death-syndrome (SIDS) and infant asthma. If you smoke while holding your baby, there is a risk of hot cigarette ash accidentally falling and burning her.

Chocolate and Spicy Foods

You may have heard from others that various foods you eat, such as chocolate or spicy foods, can affect a nursing baby. This may be true; it all depends on the mother and the baby.

Some babies are not bothered by the various foods the mother eats. Others have gas or become fussy if the mother ingests certain things. Sometimes you'll just have to experiment and see what happens.

If you find your baby extremely fussy after you eat spicy Mexican or Indian foods, for example, avoid these until after you wean your baby. Or wait until some time has passed to try it again—your baby's maturing digestive system may be able to handle some foods better as he ages.

Can Colic Result from Foods You Eat?

One study has shown that a breastfeeding mother's diet may affect whether the baby has colic. (See the discussion on page 92 for more information on colic.) Although the causes of colic are unknown at this time, certain foods have long been suspected of contributing to the problem.

The study had nursing women keep a record of their diet and corresponding fussiness in their babies. When women ate cauliflower, cabbage, broccoli, cow's milk, onions and chocolate, their babies were more colicky.

At this time, we don't recommend avoiding any foods, but we suggest you be aware if foods cause problems for your baby. The foods listed above may be ones to limit or to avoid during breastfeeding, if your baby has problems after you eat any of them.

Baby's Allergies to Some Foods

Some babies react to a food in their mother's diet, due to an allergic reaction to the food by the baby. The most common problem-causing foods are cow's milk and other dairy products. If you discover that your baby is allergic to the dairy products you consume, it can take quite a while for symptoms to improve after you eliminate the food from your diet. If you must cut out an important food from your eating plan, such as dairy products, consult a nutritionist for guidance. Your doctor can help you with this situation. The food that you must eliminate might be very important for you

Menus for Breastfeeding and Bottlefeeding Moms

On the next two pages are sample menus of the kind of foods you should eat each day, whether you choose to breastfeed or bottlefeed. Each day's plan contains a selection of nutritious food from the food groups you need during this important time. The quantity of food in these sample plans is for a woman who weighed 130 pounds (9.4 stones) before pregnancy.

If You Bottlefeed

A day's nutrition for a bottlefeeding mother is different from that of a woman who breastfeeds. You don't need to consume as many calories, and your fluid intake need not be as high.

Breakfast
½ toasted English muffin
1 T. peanut butter
4 ounces plain yogurt

Midmorning Snack
½ cup peaches, fresh or canned in water
4 ounces skim milk
1 cereal bar

Lunch
2 cups salad
2 T. light salad dressing
2 slices bread
1 slice low-fat cheese (you may wish to substitute goat's- or sheep's-milk cheeses if you have a cow's-milk allergy)
1 piece of fruit, such as an apple or pear

Midafternoon Snack
1 slice of toast
4 ounces skim milk
1 small piece of fruit

Dinner
1 small chicken breast, boiled or baked
½ cup sautéed fresh vegetables
1 slice whole-wheat bread
sliced tomatoes
1 glass water

Snack
1 cup instant fat-free cocoa
1 small cookie

If You Breastfeed

Nutrition for a nursing mother needs to be high in quality, but it needs to taste good, too! The foods listed below supply you with the nutrition you need to help you produce breast milk and to give you the energy you need while nursing.

Breakfast
1 egg, scrambled or poached
2 slices toast
1 T. margarine
½ grapefruit or cantaloupe
8 ounces skim milk

Midmorning Snack
1 cup tea
1 cup grapes
2 crackers

Lunch
2 cups salad
2 T. light salad dressing
2 slices bread
1 slice low-fat cheese (you may wish to substitute goat's- or sheep's-milk cheeses if you have or your baby has a cow's-milk allergy)
1 piece of fruit, such as an apple or a pear
8 ounces of water

Midafternoon Snack
1 slice of raisin toast
2 T. peanut butter
½ cup cottage cheese, low-fat
½ cup fruit

Dinner
1 small chicken breast, boiled or baked
1½ cups sautéed fresh vegetables
⅔ cup brown rice
sliced tomatoes
8 ounces of water

Snack
4 ounces plain yogurt
4 small crackers

CHAPTER 6

Exercise after Pregnancy

One of the most frequent questions a woman asks her doctor after her baby is born is, "How soon can I start exercising?" After months of watching their bodies change so dramatically, many women want to regain their prepregnancy figures as soon as possible. They want to get their bodies back in shape and are eager to begin exercising soon after their baby is born.

Exercise can be very important to you. It can help you feel better, as well as helping to lift your spirits. It can also increase your circulation, help you heal more quickly and ease any pains or soreness you may be feeling.

There are many things you can do to help your body get back in shape. As a matter of fact, you can start by doing simple isometric exercises right after delivery. Practice holding your stomach muscles in, or start with mild Kegel exercises (see page 67). When you go to the bathroom, try tightening your pelvic-floor and abdominal muscles; start and stop your urine stream for a good workout. Even sitting down can be an exercise—sit in a chair while tightening your pelvic-floor muscles and abdominals. Plant your feet firmly on the floor. Align your hips and shoulders while sitting straight in a chair. Open your shoulders and lengthen your neck. Keep your head high.

As soon as you are up and about, while still recovering in the hospital, you can do other forms of exercise, as long as you didn't have a C-section or any complications during the birth. Start slowly, then *gradually* increase your exercise level. When you feel able, get up and walk around in the hospital. Mild stretching of your legs and arms may feel very good after delivery. During delivery, a woman's muscles may tense during the pushing phase; stretching after recovery can relieve some of this tension.

Other exercises you can do to help you feel better soon after you have your baby include leg stretches, neck and shoulder rolls, shoulder shrugs, and foot and ankle circles. Be sure to ask your doctor or the nurses taking care of you if it's OK to do these activities.

Whatever your previous level of fitness, there should be no harm in initiating a simple stretching program soon after you are up and about, unless there are any contraindications. If you have done yoga exercises in the past, some of the gentler stretches may be good to do at this time.

Exercise is important to your feeling of well-being. If you exercised regularly during pregnancy, you may be able to accelerate your after-pregnancy program a little. Your body is probably still in good condition, so after delivery, you can begin exercising and increase your levels a little more quickly. One caution—don't expect to leave the hospital in the shape or physical condition you were in before you became pregnant. It will take a while for your stomach muscles to get back to normal.

Let your body and your healthcare providers guide you as to how much you can do and what level of intensity you can put into your exercises. Changes in your cardiovascular system from pregnancy can last for up to 6 weeks postpartum, which may affect your ability to exercise.

Exercise after a C-Section

If you have had a Cesarean delivery, exercise is very important. In the hospital, you'll probably have to practice coughing or deep breathing to keep your lungs clear. Wiggle your toes to aid circulation. Walking may not be easy, but it helps minimize the chances of developing a blood clot. Check with your doctor before starting any regular exercise routine or exercise program.

It may take you longer to get your stomach back in shape after a C-section than if you had a vaginal delivery. You may have to wait as long as 10 weeks before you can do stomach crunches, which is the best exercise for tightening stretched abdominal muscles.

Within 3 to 4 weeks, you may be able to get back into a regular exercise program. It might take longer before you can engage in activities that require all-out effort, such as running or lifting heavy weights. Full recovery could take up to 6 months.

If you experience any pain, it is essential to listen to your body. Pain may be an indication that you are not fully recovered, so you may need to ease up on your activities.

Exercising at Home

After you return home, do something you enjoy, and do it on a regular basis. You may find that as much as you want to exercise, it's very difficult to fit it into your busy schedule. Try to allow time for it so that you don't neglect physical activity. Exercise by doing some type of aerobic activity for 20 to 30 minutes at least 3 times a week (5 times a week is best for getting back in shape).

Walking and swimming are excellent exercises to help you get back in shape. Some non-weightbearing activities are excellent, such as riding a stationary bicycle or working out on a stair stepper. Even mildly aerobic exercises, such as light step aerobics or water aerobics, can be started soon after delivery. If you want to do water exercises, your doctor will probably advise you to wait until bleeding stops completely, which could take from 3 to 6 weeks.

You might want to begin strengthening exercises, using light weights, very soon after your baby's birth. Use 1- to 2-lb. weights for arm and leg exercises; use ankle weights for your legs.

Be careful about beginning an exercise program too soon. Don't overtire yourself; get adequate rest. Before you start any postpartum exercise program, be sure to check with your doctor. He or she may have some particular advice for you.

It's important to remember that getting back into shape takes time. It is easy to feel discouraged when you begin because you probably want immediate results. Understand that that won't happen, and relax. As the saying goes, "It took 9 months for your body to get into the shape it is now," and it will take some time to get it back into the shape you want.

Don't be too hard on yourself, and don't expect miracles. It may take some planning and dedication on your part to fit an exercise routine into your busy schedule and all the adjustments you are making in caring for your baby. However, you'll be happy you did when you see positive results. And you'll find you have more energy, which you probably need even more now that you have a new baby!

Ensuring Your Success

There are some things you can to do to help yourself be successful in your workouts. To lose fat, you'll want to do some type of aerobic activity, such as biking, running, swimming or aerobic-exercise classes. These exercises use large-muscle groups and will also elevate your heart rate and burn calories, which in turn burns up the fat your body stored during pregnancy. If you can work out for 20 to 40 minutes 3 to 5 times a week, you'll find your body will respond fairly quickly.

You may feel self-conscious about exercising with others, if you feel out of shape. Find a class for new mothers, or exercise with someone else who has just had a baby. Work out when traffic is light at the gym, such as late morning or early afternoon.

If you can't get away from home to exercise, an exercise videotape that you can do at home is another option. You can work out while your baby is sleeping or while your other children nap.

Tips for Starting an Exercise Program

You might also want to consider the following as you plan your exercise program.

- Before you do anything, be sure to check with your doctor about starting an exercise program. He or she may have some guidelines or suggestions for you in your particular situation. If you had a Cesarean delivery, you must be certain that your body has healed first, and you are ready to exercise safely.
- Do something you enjoy. Choose some sort of exercise that you will continue on a regular basis. If you hate running, it's probably not a good idea to choose this form of exercise as your aerobic activity.
- Time may be limited, so use it wisely. If you have the chance to do something while your baby sleeps, do it. You may rent or buy an

exercise video or develop an exercise routine you can do at home. Fit all or part of it into your schedule when you can.

- Pay attention to your nutritional needs. Don't go on a strict diet in an attempt to regain your figure quickly. You need adequate nutrition to make breast milk, if you breastfeed. Even if you don't breastfeed, your body needs energy to take care of your baby and yourself, so don't skimp on your food. Eat nutritiously, and accept the fact it may take you a little longer than you would like to get back in shape. That's OK—it's for the good of you and your baby. See the previous chapter for advice on nutrition.

- Don't compare yourself with anyone else—even your prepregnancy self! Your body has undergone some major changes, so don't be too hard on yourself. It may take longer than you expect to lose weight, and you may find your body shape has changed because of the pregnancy. You may have to accept these changes because there may not be much you can do about them. Avoid weighing yourself on the scales. Instead, let your clothes be your guide. Tune in to your body—see how you feel. Use these measures as a gauge to determine your progress.

- Work out with a friend, especially another new mom. Walk together or agree to do some other type of activity. Take your babies when possible. If you know someone else depends on you for support, it may be easier to stay committed.

- If you find you're getting bored with your routine or you feel very tired, try to make some positive changes, such as experimenting with other activities. Keep at it, even when you feel exhausted— sometimes exercise can help increase your energy level and will help you feel less tired as you get going.

- Be sure you always warm up and cool down, whether you are doing aerobic exercise or toning exercises. Warm up by walking briskly or marching in place for 5 to 10 minutes. When finished with your activities, cool down by stretching for at least 5 minutes.

Before you begin exercising, you'll probably need to gather together some things to help make your workout easier and more enjoyable. Paying attention to these details before you begin will increase the enjoyment and benefits you receive from your exercise program.

Wear the right clothes and shoes. Clothes should be comfortable and allow your body to "breathe." Wear shoes that offer good support. A sports bra may provide added relief to enlarged and sore breasts.

Drink lots of water. Start before you exercise, and keep well hydrated throughout your exercise period.

Exercises to Tone Your Body

In this section, you will find a collection of various *isometric* and *isotonic* exercises you can do to help you get back in shape. *Isometric* exercises pit one muscle or part of the body against another or against an immovable object, such as a wall, in a strong, motionless action. These activities include pressing, pulling or pushing. *Isotonic* exercises tense the muscles against a heavy or resistant force; they help build muscle strength. These activities include weight lifting.

This section includes both isometric and isotonic exercises to help you build or regain strength in your muscles. *Aerobic* exercise should be pursued in addition to these activities because aerobic exercise increases the body's metabolism and helps burn fat.

In addition to doing some sort of aerobic exercise, choose exercises from this section that focus on body areas you need to work on. Try to do these activities at least three times a week—every other day helps tone muscles. You might want to alternate aerobic activity and toning exercises from one day to the next.

You may notice that many of these exercises are for toning tummy muscles. We have found that this area is the one many new mothers are most concerned about, so we have included quite a few for you to choose from.

Kegel Exercises
This exercise is one of the best you can do to help tighten your pelvic-floor muscles. It's very helpful in getting your vaginal muscles in shape after the delivery and can be done anywhere and any time.

First, tighten, then release, your lower-pelvis muscles. Then tighten the muscles higher in the pelvis until you reach those at the top. Hold for a count of 10, then release slowly. Repeat 3 or 4 times.
—*Good for toning pelvic-floor muscles.*

Your Other Pelvic-Floor-Muscle Strengthener
Lie on the floor on your back as shown in the illustration below. Place arms straight out from your sides. Cross one leg over the opposite ankle, and squeeze legs together. Hold 4 seconds, then release. Repeat with your legs crossed the opposite way. Do 6 times for each side.
—*Good for toning pelvic-floor muscles.*

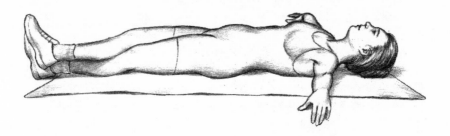

Leg-and-Back Stretch

Place a chair in the corner of the room so that it won't slide when you push against it. Place your right foot on the chair seat; support yourself against the wall with your hand, if necessary. Stretch your right leg behind you, then lift your chest and arch your back. Turn your shoulders and lean your torso to the right. Hold for 25 to 30 seconds. Do three stretches for each side. Do this stretch before beginning abdominal exercises.

—*Good for toning legs and back muscles.*

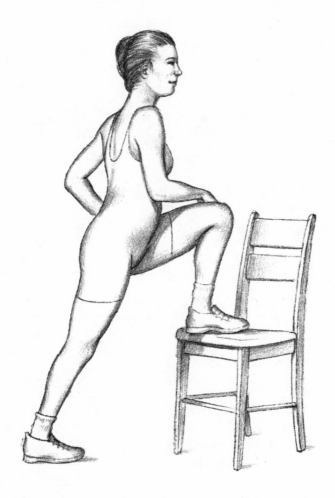

Tummy Tightener

Lie on the floor. Lift both feet about 18 inches off the floor, bending your knees at a right angle. Place your hands under your hips to support your lower back. Raise your head slightly, keeping your shoulders and upper back on floor. Bring the knees toward your face while lifting your feet. Use abdominal muscles to lift your legs; don't push against the floor with your arms. Hold for a count of 5. Begin by doing 3 and work up to 25.

—*Good for toning tummy muscles.*

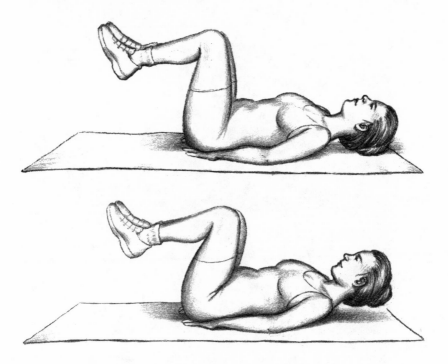

Lower-Belly Tightener

Lie on your back on the floor, with your hands at your sides. Hold feet together, bend your knees and lift your legs up to a 90-degree angle. Using your lower abdominals, and making sure not to push with your hands, lift your hips up a few inches, hold, then release. Gradually work up to 15 repetitions each day.

—*Good for toning tummy muscles.*

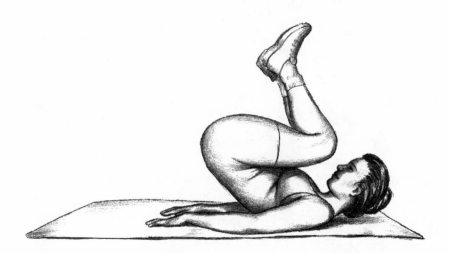

Stretches for Relief of a Tense Back

To ease a tense back, sit on the edge of a chair, with your knees 6 inches apart and your feet facing forward. Lean forward until your tummy touches your thighs. Clasp your wrists together under your thighs. Breathe deeply through your nose, and let your chin drop onto your chest. Hold for 30 seconds, then push back to an upright sitting position. Repeat 3 or 4 times.

—*Good for easing tight back muscles.*

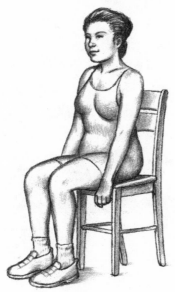

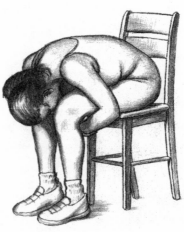

Arm-and-Shoulder Stretches

Sit up straight. Lace your fingers together behind your head, keeping elbows apart. Inhale and push your interlaced hands, with your fingers still together, toward the ceiling. Exhale and return your hands to their position behind your head.

—*Good for toning arms and shoulder muscles.*

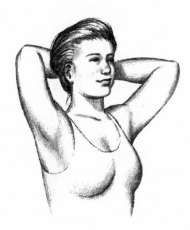

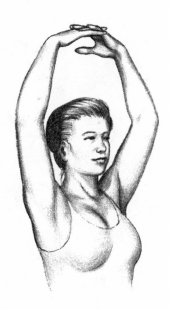

Leg Stretches

Stand with your feet wider than shoulder width apart. Turn your toes out slightly. Place your hands on your waist, and squat with your knees over your toes. Hold for count of 3. Keeping your back straight, slowly raise your body to a standing position. Repeat 8 times.

—*Good for toning leg muscles.*

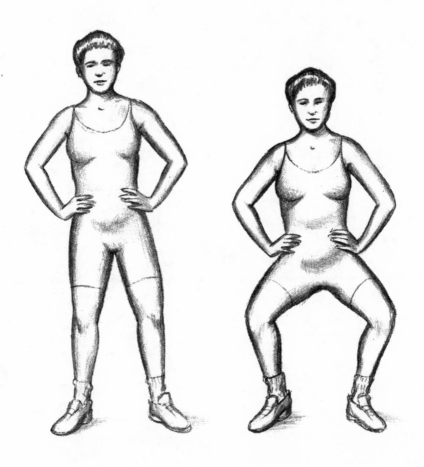

Reverse Curls (also called *Pelvic Tilts*)

Lie flat on your back with your knees drawn up so your feet are flat on the floor. Place your hands by your sides, keeping your shoulders on the floor. Squeezing your buttock muscles together, lift your hips from the floor high enough so that you create a straight line between your hips, knees and shoulders. Hold for a count of 5, then slowly return your hips to the floor. Repeat 5 times.

—*Good for toning tummy muscles.*

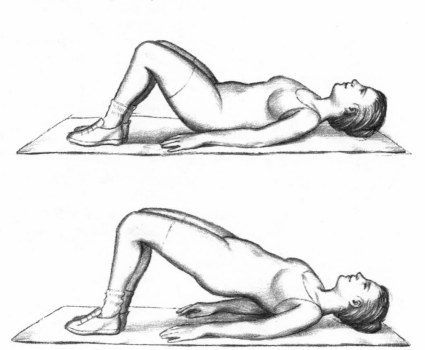

Tummy Compressions

Like Kegel exercises, you can do this just about anywhere. Standing or sitting, take a deep breath and inhale. While exhaling, tighten your tummy muscles as though you were zipping up a pair of tight jeans. Repeat 6 or 8 times.

—*Good for toning tummy muscles.*

Tummy Crunches

Lying on the floor, bend your knees with your feet flat on the floor. Place your hands behind your head. Tighten your tummy muscles as you lift your head and shoulders slightly. Keep your chin open (look forward and up). Hold the crunch for 4 seconds. Repeat 5 times.

—*Good for toning tummy muscles.*

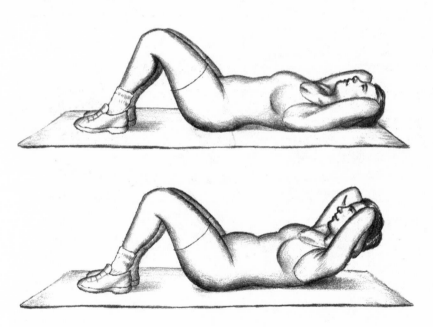

Side Crunches
To work the sides of your abdomen, position yourself as for the basic tummy crunch. After you lift, rotate toward one knee. Hold the crunch for 4 seconds, then repeat for the other side. Repeat 5 times.
—*Good for tightening oblique muscles (muscles on the sides of your waist).*

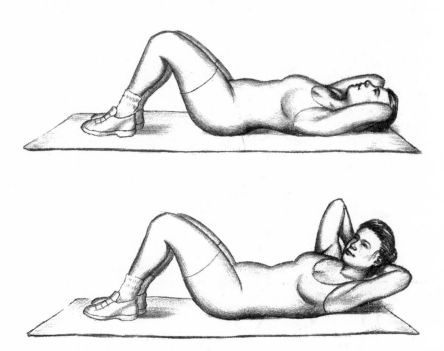

Breast Boosters

Sit on the edge of a chair. Using light weights (2 to 3 lbs. each) to start, raise your arms to shoulder level, and bend your elbows so that your hands point toward the ceiling. Slowly bring your elbows and arms together in front of your face. Hold for 4 seconds, then slowly open to shoulder width. Repeat 8 times, and progress up to 20 times.
—*Good for tightening breasts muscles, to keep breasts from sagging.*

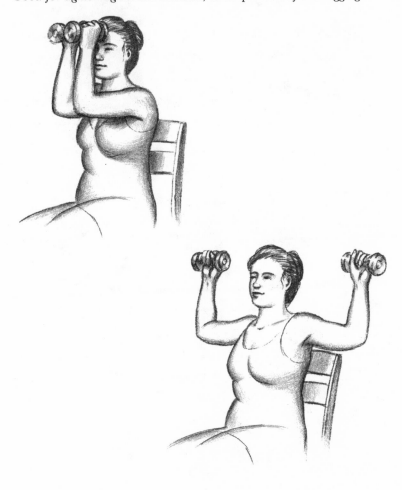

Pushups

Kneel on the floor, putting your weight on your hands and knees. Bending your elbows, lower your chest toward the floor while inhaling, until you are about 2 inches from the floor. Hold for a count of 2. Straighten your arms and push back up while exhaling. Hold for a count of 3. Repeat 6 times.

—*Good for strengthening arm and back muscles.*

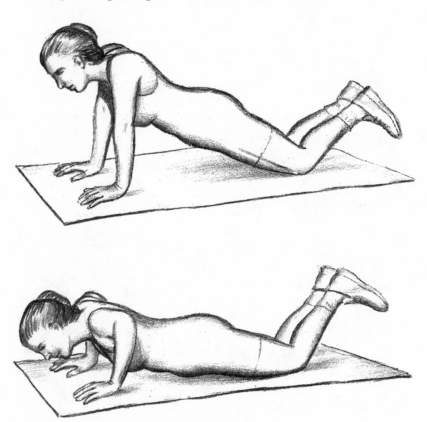

Waist Toner

Stand with your feet apart and your knees relaxed. Holding a light weight in your right hand (an unopened 16-ounce can will do fine), extend your right arm straight over your head. Contract your tummy muscles while bending slightly at the waist, then swing your arm down and over your left foot. Complete the exercise by returning your arm to its original position above your right shoulder. Repeat 8 times on each side.

—*Good for slimming your waistline.*

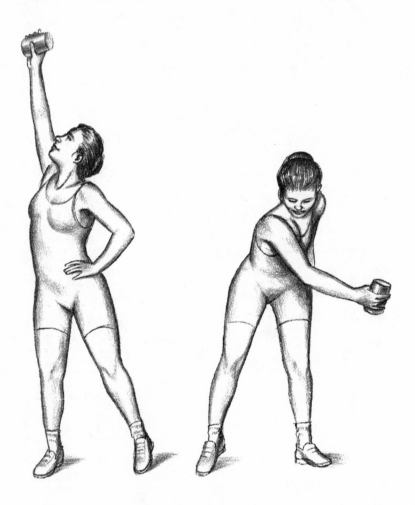

Leg Lifts

Sit on the edge of a chair, and place both feet flat on the floor. Relax your shoulders and curve your arms over your head. Keeping your back straight, hold in abdominal muscles while you extend one leg out in front of you. Using your thigh muscles only, lift the leg about 10 inches off the floor. Hold for a count of 5, then slowly lower your foot. Repeat 10 times with each leg.

—*Good for toning thigh muscles, hips and buttocks.*

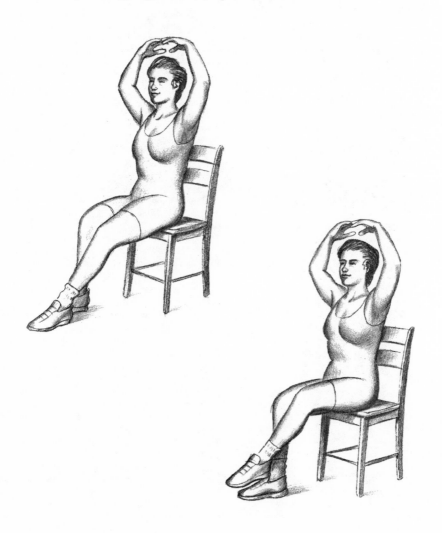

Spinal Extensions

Lie on your tummy with your right hand under your forehead. Stretch your left hand out in front of you. Slowly lift your left hand and right leg off the floor at the same time. Hold for a count of 2, then lower slowly. Repeat 8 times for each side.

—*Good for strengthening back muscles and toning tummy muscles.*

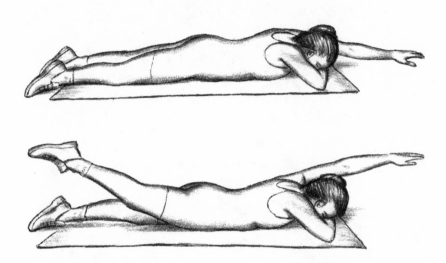

Side Leg Lifts
Hold onto a door jamb or the back of a sturdy chair. Beginning with
your left leg, point your toe and lift your leg forward, up to 90 degrees,
then lower your leg to the floor. Without stopping, lift the same leg to
the side, as far as you can, but not beyond 90 degrees. Return the leg
to your starting position. Repeat 10 times for each leg.
—*Good for toning leg muscles and buttocks.*

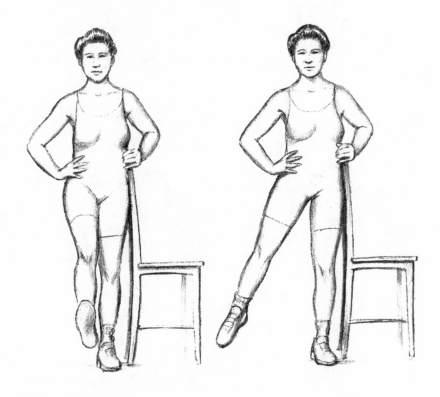

Upper-Chest Stretch

To help your posture, stand or sit on the floor, and clasp your hands behind you. Lift your arms until you feel a good stretch in your upper-chest area and upper arms. Hold for a count of 5, then lower your arms. Repeat 8 times.

—*Good for stretching arm and back muscles.*

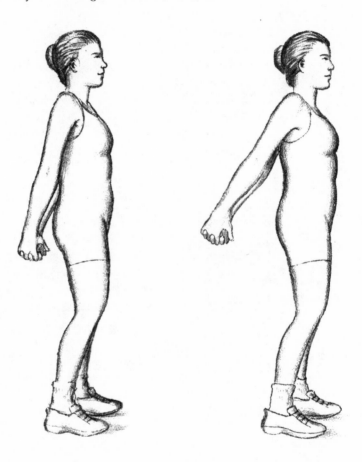

Double Leg Lifts
Lie on your back on the floor. Keeping both legs together, lift your legs slowly from the hip. Be sure you use your tummy muscles for this one. Hold for 6 seconds, then slowly lower both legs to the floor. Repeat, gradually building up to 8 repetitions.
—*Good for toning tummy muscles.*

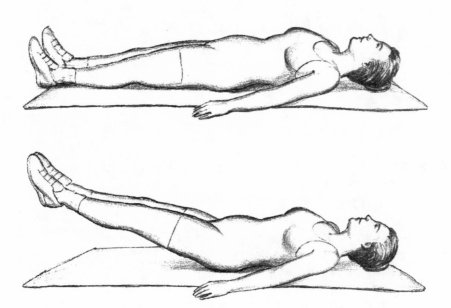

CHAPTER 7

Adjusting to Life with Your New Baby

You have looked forward for many months to welcoming your new baby into your life. It is exciting to bond together into a family. However, during your first few days and weeks at home, you may begin to wonder if all your baby will ever do is eat, sleep and make a mess in her pants! You may wonder if she will ever get on any type of schedule.

This can be a time of stress for everyone in your family. It might work out better if you don't try to put you or your baby on a rigid schedule. It's better if you can let a schedule develop in a more flexible, natural fashion. You'll probably find this is more convenient, and you'll be able to make changes gradually as your baby grows and develops.

You may find your baby seems to need much more sleep than other babies. It is quite normal for some babies to get day and night mixed up for a while. Take heart—this doesn't usually last longer than a few weeks. If possible, keep your baby awake and active during the day; it may help him to get on a more-regular sleep schedule.

In the first 4 weeks of life, your baby may sleep as long as 20 hours a day. You may wonder if he will ever be awake long enough to get to know him. He may seldom be awake for longer than 25 to 30 minutes at a time. And it is during this time that you will feed, change and bathe him. Use this time to cuddle and bond—you will see that each day he will become more aware of you and his surroundings.

Babies feed quite often in the first few months of life, whether they are breastfed or bottlefed. A baby can feed every 2 to 4 hours. When your baby is quite young, feed her whenever she's hungry—don't try to establish any schedule. Denying your baby food when she is hungry can cause her to become anxious. If you breastfeed, note each time you breastfeed and for how long. If you bottlefeed, note when your baby feeds and how much she consumes. This is important information to share with your pediatrician on your baby's first visit.

It's surprising to find out how often a baby needs to be changed! A baby may wet his diaper every 2 to 4 hours, and the number of bowel movements varies from one baby to the next. If you breastfeed, your baby may have a bowel movement only once every couple of days; this is normal. If you bottlefeed, your baby may have as many as six bowel movements a day, usually following a feeding. This, too, is normal.

Change your baby as soon as possible. Babies have very delicate skin, and wet diapers can lead to diaper rash. If your baby has diaper rash already, a wet diaper can make it worse. And it hurts! In the beginning, you may need as many as 100 diapers a week. As your baby grows older, this number will diminish.

It's also normal for your baby to cry. A baby cries to make his wants known—he has no other way of communicating with you. Some babies cry more than others. You will soon learn how to distinguish different cries in your baby—you'll be able to tell a "hungry cry" from a "lonely cry" or a "bored cry." It just takes time and practice. Until you learn what different cries mean, check the baby's diapers, try burping him again and be sure the baby is not uncomfortable. Sometimes your baby just wants to be held and cuddled by you.

Beginning Life with Your New Baby

Your baby is a precious creation—you must handle her with care. Your newborn lacks muscle control, so you'll need to take precautions to make sure you hold her correctly. It also helps to hold your baby in the correct positions because she tends to become startled as a result of sudden changes. Holding her correctly can avoid injury and yelps of fright. Try the following:

- always keep your hand behind your baby's head when you lift him or hold him at your shoulder

- when carrying him in your arms, his head will probably extend beyond your elbow—be careful not to bump his head against the doorway or wall
- lift your baby slowly
- don't rush when you carry him
- don't move your baby too suddenly

Every parent has probably been overprotective at times with a new baby. You may dress your baby too warmly or keep her isolated from everyone else to avoid germs or check on her 10 times a night.

It's OK to be cautious, but relax. Your baby needs to be exposed to people; you can't keep all infections away from her—it isn't possible. However, it's probably best to avoid crowds, like those at malls or markets, at least during her first month.

Keep your home temperature comfortable, and dress your baby comfortably. It is unnecessary to keep your home "tropical." As a matter of fact, it could be detrimental for *everyone* in the family if you do this. Generally, 68°F (20°C) to 70°F (21°C) is a good range. Don't assume a baby is cold just because his hands and feet are. The best indicator is your baby's mood. If you can't comfort your baby by holding or feeding him, he may be too hot or too cold.

When you do take your baby out, be sure you dress him appropriately. Keep him out of the wind and the sun, too. Layers work best—add one more layer than you have on, or add a light blanket. Babies lose heat through their hands, feet and scalp (as do adults), so be sure all three areas are well covered in cold weather.

While sunscreens can work wonders for you, don't use them on a baby younger than 6 months. They can be very irritating to delicate skin. Put a hat and protective clothing on the baby for even a brief outing in the sun, especially in very hot, sunny areas.

You don't have to walk on tiptoes around your little one—this isn't practical. The usual household noises won't harm your baby; being exposed to them will make her less sensitive, and she'll have an easier time sleeping if she's used to some of the background noises in your home.

What Does Your Baby Look Like?

Many parents are surprised, then somewhat dismayed, by how their baby looks. Don't feel upset if this happens. Immediately after the birth, your baby may not be the beautiful child he or she will become in a short time.

Your baby is born wet, usually with some blood on his body. A white or yellow waxy substance, called *vernix*, may cover part or much of his body. This is easily removed by cleaning the baby's skin.

You will probably notice that your baby's head is large in proportion to the rest of her body. It can look enormous on the baby's tiny body. At birth, the head measures 25% of her entire length. As she grows, this will change until her head is only about 12% of her adult height.

If your baby made his appearance into this world through the birth canal, his head may be misshapen or elongated. This shape is only temporary, and its appearance becomes more normal over the next few days.

You may notice other oddities in your baby's appearance. Her cheeks may be pouchy, her eyelids swollen and her head pointy. A newborn's nose may look too flat to breathe through, but babies do manage to breathe through their noses.

You may be distressed when you see the baby's pulse throbbing at the two soft spots on her head, called the *fontanels*. Don't worry about it.

Your baby may be born with lots of hair or none at all. If she has an abundance of hair, this first hair usually falls out in the first 6 months and is later replaced by hair that may be entirely different in color and texture. If she's bald, it's not a permanent condition; her hair will eventually grow.

A newborn's eyes may be swollen or puffy immediately following birth, but it subsides in a few days. This is caused by the pressure in the birth canal. You may also notice your baby's eyes are slightly irritated and red. This results from the drops or ointment applied to his eyes shortly after birth to prevent eye infections. Irritation and redness usually disappear within a couple of days.

One of your baby's eyes may wander when she looks at you, or she may look cross-eyed. Don't let this concern you. Her eye muscles aren't strong enough yet to control her eye movements. A wandering eye usually corrects itself by the time the baby is 6 months old. If she still has a problem after that, discuss it with your healthcare provider.

The skinfolds at the inner corners of a baby's eyes can make it look as if the baby is squinting. As time passes, these folds become less prominent, and your baby will no longer look as if he's squinting.

A baby's skin may appear wrinkled, peeling, scratched, blotchy, hairy or pimpled, or it may look perfect. It often begins to dry out and may become flaky and scaly after birth. This condition can last for a few weeks. You don't need to treat it, but you may want to rub a little lotion into your baby's skin.

If you are worried that your baby has been born with a disability or deformity, talk to your pediatrician about your concerns. If a problem is diagnosed, remember that you do not have to cope alone; ask your pediatrician about the support groups and specialist organizations that are available to help.

When Your Baby Cries

Most parents express their distress when they hear their baby cry—especially when they cannot comfort the baby. Crying is natural for babies; it's their way of communicating. When your baby cries, he is communicating to you that he is hungry, tired or lonely. Or he may be telling you he needs to be burped or changed. He might cry if he feels sick, scared or in pain. Sometimes a baby cries when he is overstimulated. It may seem impossible in the first few weeks of your baby's life, but you will soon learn to interpret his different cries.

It's important for you to know that the way you hold your baby brings special comfort to her. When you touch her, it tells her she is not alone. You won't spoil her if you comfort her when she is fussy. Finding the tricks that work with your baby may only come through trial and error, but you'll eventually learn what works best for her. Some common solutions include reducing stimulation, giving the baby something to comfort her, such as her hand or a pacifier, wrapping your baby securely in a blanket, laying your baby on her stomach across your lap and stroking her, or softly humming or singing to her.

It's important for you to realize that occasionally your baby's crying may cause you distress. If you find this happening, ask a friend or relative to stay with the baby so you can take a break. Get out of the house for a walk or for some personal quiet time. Exercise can help relieve any stress you may feel (see Chapter 6).

Your Baby's Health

It's inevitable—your baby will get sick sometime. Whether it's a cold, an ear infection, colic or something else, you need to be prepared. If your baby exhibits any of the following symptoms, call your doctor:

- fever higher than 101°F (38.3°C)
- inconsolable crying for long periods of time
- problems with urination
- projectile vomiting, in which a baby's stomach contents can come out with great force
- the baby appears lethargic or floppy when held
- severe diarrhea
- unusual behavior
- poor appetite

Any of these could be an indication your baby is ill.

Dehydration
Dehydration in an infant can be very serious. If it occurs, call your healthcare provider immediately. There are some warning signs to watch for.

Warning Signs of Dehydration in a Baby

- The baby wets fewer than six cloth or five disposable diapers a day.
- The baby's urine is dark yellow or orange; it should be pale yellow.
- The baby has fewer than two loose stools a day.
- The baby seems to be having trouble sucking.
- The soft spot on the baby's head is sunken in.
- The baby is listless or otherwise unhealthy.

If you are concerned, call your doctor. A change in the number of diapers used or the consistency of the bowel movement may be the first clue.

Diarrhea
Your baby may experience diarrhea—it's not uncommon for this to occur. He'll need extra water and minerals to prevent dehydration. Your doctor may recommend an oral electrolyte solution to help replenish your baby's lost fluids and minerals.

Ear infections
It may be difficult for you to determine that your baby has an ear infection. Symptoms that may indicate an ear infection in babies less than 6 months of age include irritability that lasts all day, sleeplessness, lethargy and feeding difficulties. These symptoms may be hard to discern and may not be accompanied by a fever. For babies between 6 and 12 months of age, the symptoms are similar, except that a fever is more common. The onset of ear pain may be sudden, acute and more noticeable.

Jaundice
Jaundice is the yellow staining of the skin, sclera (eyes) and deeper tissues of the body. The baby looks yellow because excess amounts of *bilirubin*, a chemical produced in the liver, have accumulated in the baby's blood, and the baby is unable to handle it.

Jaundice is caused by too much bilirubin in the baby's blood, a condition called *hyperbilirubinemia*. It can be dangerous for the baby if left untreated.

If your baby's pediatrician and the nurses in the baby nursery suspect that your baby has jaundice, she will be kept under observation. They will determine what type of treatment is necessary.

Phototherapy is used to treat jaundice. The baby is placed under special lights, which penetrate his skin and destroy the bilirubin. In some parts of the world, special lights may not be necessary. To treat the jaundice, the baby is placed outside in the sunshine for very short periods of time; the sunlight destroys the excess bilirubin. In more severe cases, blood-exchange transfusions may be necessary.

Colic
Colic is a condition marked by episodes of loud, sudden crying and fussiness, which can often last for hours. About 20% of all babies experience this unexplained pain and crying. In full-blown colic, the baby's abdomen becomes distended, and the infant passes gas frequently.

The only way to know if your baby has colic is to visit your pediatrician or family physician. He or she can determine if it is colic or if your baby is having some other problem.

Colic usually appears gradually in the infant about 2 weeks after birth. As time passes, the condition may worsen; however, it often disappears around the age of 3 months, but occasionally lasts until the baby is 4 months old. Colic attacks usually occur at night, beginning in the late afternoon and early evening, and can last as long as 3 to 4 hours. However, such attacks cease as quickly as they begin.

Researchers have been studying colic and its causes for a long time, but we still have little exact evidence of why it occurs. Theories about its causes include:

- immaturity of the digestive system
- intolerance to cow's-milk protein in formula or breast milk
- fatigue in the infant

At this time, we cannot offer a definitive treatment that will effectively end colic. Most doctors recommend using a variety of methods to try to ease the baby's discomfort.

Tips for Treating Colic

- Offer the baby your breast or a bottle of formula.
- Try noncow's-milk formula, if you bottlefeed.
- Carry your baby in a sling during an attack. Motion and closeness often help.
- Try using a pacifier to soothe the baby.
- Put the baby on her stomach across your knees, and rub her back.
- Wrap the baby snugly in a blanket.
- Massage or stroke the baby's tummy.

Your Baby's Sleeping Habits

As we've already stated, your baby will spend a lot of time sleeping in the first few months. Sleeping is very important for a baby, and you'll soon realize what kind of sleep schedule is best for your infant. The wisest thing you can do as a parent is to establish a routine to help your baby develop healthy sleeping habits. The list below may give you some helpful hints on how to do this.

Hints on Helping Your Baby to Sleep

- Wait until your baby is tired before putting him to bed.
- Develop a regular, predictable routine for bedtime.
- Develop good sleep associations, such as a favorite blanket or toy, or a pacifier. Whatever you do, don't put your baby to bed with a bottle!
- Never leave your baby alone on a waterbed.
- Limit daytime naps to a few hours each.
- Don't overstimulate the baby when you get up for nighttime feedings.
- By day, let your baby nap in a sunlit area or in a room with some lights on, with some background noise. At night, put your baby in a dark, quiet room to sleep.
- Keep your baby up during the day by talking and singing or by providing other stimulation.

Research has proved that it is better to place a baby on his side or back when putting him down to sleep. We have discovered that this position greatly reduces the incidence of SIDS (sudden-infant-death syndrome). Other safe sleeping tips include making sure the mattress is safe and in good repair. Crib slats should be no farther apart than $2^3/8$ inches (6 cm). Don't use comforters, pillows or cushions that are soft and have loosely filled surfaces—these could interfere with your baby's breathing. Avoid a waterbed mattress for a baby because the baby may become trapped and suffocate.

Sleep patterns develop differently for bottlefed and breastfed babies. Bottlefed babies sleep longer at night as they mature. Breastfed infants don't shift to longer sleep patterns until around the time they are weaned.

Taking Care of Your Baby

Your baby's umbilical-cord stump will fall off 7 to 10 days after birth. Until it does, clean your baby with sponge baths instead of tub baths.

Cleaning Your Baby's Eyes, Nose and Ears
To remove sleep from your baby's eyes, use a moistened cotton ball. Place the cotton ball at the inner corner of the eye, and wipe vertically down the nose.

Never put anything inside your baby's nose. If you need to remove dried nasal secretions, gently wipe around the nose. Dried nasal secretions are usually sneezed out.

Never probe in your baby's ears with any object! Earwax is there for a purpose. It's OK to clean around the outside of the ears with a soft washcloth, but don't insert anything inside your baby's ears.

Diapers

You will probably have to decide between cloth and disposable diapers. What you choose depends on your lifestyle, your budget and your baby. Disposable diapers are very convenient because you don't need pins or plastic pants, and they don't need to be washed. On the other hand, cloth diapers can be reused many times. Some styles don't need pins or plastic pants. You will need adequate washing and drying facilities, or you may choose a diaper service. Many people use a combination of disposable and cloth diapers.

Car Restraints—For the Safety of Your Baby

Every time your baby rides in the car, he should be in an approved safety-restraint seat. In an accident, an unrestrained child becomes a missilelike object in a car. The force of a crash can literally pull a child out of an adult's arms!

It's incredible, but one study showed that more than 30 deaths a year occur due to infants being unrestrained in a car while going home from the hospital after birth! In nearly all of these cases, if the baby had been in an approved infant-restraint system, he or she would have survived the accident. Don't take chances—keep your baby safely restrained.

Many states now have laws that govern safety-restraint systems. Call your local hospital or police department, and ask for information. Some hospitals won't let you take the baby home if he or she is not going to ride in an approved safety-restraint seat. Many hospitals have loaners you can borrow until you get your own.

The safest spot in a car is in the middle of the back seat. In this position, your baby will be more protected in the event of a side collision. Manufacturers recommend not putting the car seat in the front seat if you have a passenger-side airbag. If the bag inflates, it can knock the car seat around or even injure the baby.

Making Your Home Safe for Baby

It's important to make your home safe for your new baby. You may not think this is important when your baby is so small, but it is. There are many things you can do to protect your baby from the first day you bring him home.

You cannot completely baby-proof your house, but you can improve its safety. Accidents can and do (and will!) happen, so it's a good idea to make your baby's environment as safe as you possibly can. Keep in mind the following.

Tips for Safety in the Home

- Crib slats should be no farther apart than $2^3/_8$ inches (6 cm).
- Be sure the mattress fits securely.
- Keep the crib away from windows, wall decorations, heating units, climbable furniture, blind and drapery cords, and other possible dangers.
- Never use a pillow in a crib.
- Keep the dropside up and locked when baby is in the crib.
- Keep mobiles and other crib toys out of baby's reach. You may have to remove them as baby grows older.
- Never hang a pacifier or any other object around your baby's neck.
- Never leave a baby alone in the water, even if it's only a few inches deep. A baby can drown in as little as 1 inch of water.
- Never leave your baby unattended on a sofa, chair, changing table or any other surface above the floor.
- Never put an infant seat on the counter or a table.
- Always use any safety straps with baby equipment.
- Never hold your baby while you're cooking, drinking a hot beverage or smoking a cigarette.
- If you warm formula or heat baby food in the microwave, shake the bottle or stir the food before serving to avoid any hot spots.
- Don't hang anything on stroller handles; the extra weight could cause the stroller to tip over.
- Always put your baby in a car seat, even for a 2-block ride. Be sure the car seat meets federal safety guidelines and is properly installed.
- Keep stairs and other areas well lit.
- Use nonslip mats in the tub and on the bathroom floor to help prevent falls.
- Install antiscald devices in tubs and showers.

CHAPTER 8

Your Partner Is a New Parent, Too

This is a remarkable time as you begin to share the joys and responsibilities of parenting with your partner, a time of wonder and concern for both of you.

You will both have many concerns. As a mother, you probably want to be the best mother ever. Your partner also wants to be the best father he can be, and he may be wondering how his role as a parent will develop. You both may have many other questions, including those below.

Common Parenting Questions You May Have

- Will we be good parents?
- Will my partner be a good father or mother?
- Will my partner support me and help me with the very important task of parenting?
- How will my partner help me with the baby?
- What can I do to help my partner be the best father or mother he or she can be?

We will try to answer these and many other questions, some of which you may not even know you have, in this chapter. Whether you find the specific answers you seek, it is our hope that you will discover ways to help each other be good parents. Parenting may be the hardest job you will ever undertake, but it is also the most rewarding. Being able to help each other out can make the job easier and more satisfying for both of you.

(Authors' note: In this chapter, we address information to both parents. In one section we may be talking to the new mom, in another, the new dad. In a few sections, we offer information for you both. We will alert you at the beginning of each section as to which parent the particular information is directed.)

Help Your Partner Begin to Parent

(For the New Mother)

Before a man becomes a father, much of who he is is defined by his work. After his child is born, that often changes—he is now a father, and that is how he now defines himself. All else is secondary. It is important to encourage and to help your partner in his transition to fatherhood.

When a man helps care for his baby from birth, he will continue to be involved in the parenting of his child as the child grows up. One way your partner can become fully involved with his new baby is for you to help him prepare for the task.

You can begin this preparation before the birth of the baby. Childbirth classes and other prenatal preparation classes introduce dads-to-be to many aspects of childcare and parenting.

Encourage your partner to take time off from work after the baby's birth. He may have to arrange this ahead of time, so try to plan for it before the baby is born. (See the discussion of paternity leave on page 106.) Staying home for a full week after the baby is born is a good amount of time but in many cases may not be possible. As a new father, your partner may be able to make arrangements to spend more time with you and your new family member. This allows him to have enough time to get to know his baby and to become comfortable in his new role as parent.

Even if you are breastfeeding, try to share your feeding responsibilities. Expressing your milk for your partner to feed the baby can help the father and baby to bond; it can also provide a welcome respite for you. If your partner wants to give the baby a bottle of breast milk during the night, it allows you a longer period of uninterrupted sleep. You might really enjoy (and need) the sleep in the first few weeks of motherhood.

Divide tasks in the most logical way you can. If you need to rest before you start making dinner, perhaps dad can tend the baby for an hour to give you a break. Then you can prepare the dinner when you have more energy.

Trust your partner in his ability to care for your baby. Allow him the opportunity to be a good parent. Don't stand over him and correct him as he does everything—although he'll probably make some mistakes, babies are pretty resilient. Your baby may even be able to handle mistakes more easily than you! Giving your partner the space to develop his own parenting style helps him to become more confident as a parent.

Bonding with the Baby

(For the New Father)

Women are so much more fortunate than a man in that they have 9 months to bond with their baby before it is born. A father needs time to bond with his newborn, but he can begin by holding the baby as soon as the baby is born. Some suggest that a father-to-be can begin to feel bonded to his baby before the delivery by placing his hands on the mother-to-be's tummy and feeling the baby move inside the uterus. While it's important for mothers and babies to bond together, it is equally important for a man to bond with his child. Bonding allows you to connect physically and emotionally with your baby. It doesn't happen instantly, and it isn't a one-time event. But it is one of the most-important things you can do with your baby, and it helps you feel as though your baby is really your own flesh and blood.

Holding the baby, gazing into his eyes and cooing at him will help you to bond with your baby. Stroking and rubbing the baby while making eye contact heightens the sense of bonding. Babies readily respond to the human voice; talking and singing to him help strengthen the baby's connection to his parents.

It's important for you to spend time alone with your baby soon after the birth. This strengthens the feelings of attachment between you and your baby. Take your baby with you on errands, or just have her close as you go through your day. You may want to use a baby snuggler that you can wear on your chest. Just hearing your voice, smelling your scent and being physically close will help both of you become closer to one another.

Don't be afraid to ask for help and guidance if you need it. No one is an expert immediately—not even your partner! It doesn't diminish you in any way to ask others for guidance. As a matter of fact, they will admire you for having the courage to know you need assistance and being confident enough to ask for it.

Talk to other parents, especially other fathers, about your concerns. Many have had the same experiences and have shared the same feelings of doubt. The solutions and guidance they offer for some of the problems you may have can save you from future worry and hassles. As your feelings of confidence increase, your bond with your new baby will also become stronger.

Some techniques fathers have used to bond with their baby include the following activities. Try them all as you begin to build your relationship with your child.

Techniques for Bonding for Fathers

- Lie on your side on the bed. Lay baby on his side facing you. Pull him close so that he can feel your breath on his face. Sing or talk to him as you rub or stroke his body.
- Hold your baby so her head snuggles under your chin. (Be sure you have shaved recently, so you don't give her whisker burn!) Sway from side to side, and coo or sing to her. She will feel your warm breath as you exhale.
- Lay your baby on his stomach along your forearm. With your hand, support his head and chin. Let his legs hang down on either side of your arm. Carry him in this position, or sit in a chair together. Be sure to protect his head if you move around carrying him like this.
- Lie on the bed with your baby. Have your shirt off, and lay your naked (or diapered) baby against your bare skin. (This is one of the recommended bonding positions for moms as soon baby is born.) Turn your baby's head to the side so she can hear your heartbeat. Relax together, and enjoy the closeness.

Your Changing Relationship

(For the New Mother)

Your partner may feel his relationship with you is changing greatly. He may begin to look at you as the mother of his child, which can be a great change in his perception. Sometimes a man feels unnerved because he feels greater responsibility—for you and the new baby.

He may feel left out because the bond between mother and child is so strong. He may feel ignored because his partner is now so involved with the new baby. He may be hesitant to interact fully with his child because he doesn't feel confident that he can do it well. He may feel fearful that he won't be able to measure up to his new responsibilities.

These, and many other feelings, are natural. It's important for you to deal effectively with your feelings. The three "Cs" are important in this process—Communication, Compromise and Cooperation. It may be hard to start a dialogue, but you can begin by sharing your own feelings about the situation. Be specific about what you're feeling; you'll encourage him to be specific about his feelings. Open communication can help you both. Discuss issues as they arise so you can deal with them then. Be honest about your feelings and concerns.

There are other ways to help your partner move into fatherhood after the baby arrives. Educate him about childcare; you can learn together. Share books and articles about the many aspects of parenthood that you both probably have questions about.

Help the new dad become an expert at some aspect of baby care. The more a person feels in control of a situation, the more he or she is willing to participate in it. For example, let your partner bathe the baby when possible. Let him develop his own routine and control it. He may not do what you would, but as long as the baby is clean (and of course, safe), what does it matter if he doesn't do it the same way you do?

Be positive and encouraging. Everyone needs to know they're doing a good job and their efforts are appreciated. When he makes a mistake, accept it, provide as little correction as possible, praise what he has accomplished and move on.

Make things as easy as possible for your partner when he begins a new task or chore. As he becomes more adept at it, he can work out the details for himself. If he has your help and support from the beginning, he'll be more willing to pursue an activity than if he is just thrown into the task with little or no preparation.

How to Keep the Closeness in Your Relationship

(For Both the New Mother and the New Father)

With a new baby in the house, time tends to be a precious commodity, and sometimes kindness, respect and thoughtfulness go out the window. It's important to work at your relationship with your partner. You're both in this parenthood thing together, and it's more rewarding for you both if you are able to grow closer through the added responsibilities, instead of letting them separate you. There are many ways you can be kind to one another. For example, remember to involve him after the delivery. Ask him to make some of the phone calls to tell friends and family of the joyous event. Work together, and you may be surprised how strong your relationship becomes. A stronger relationship between the two of you provides security for your child.

The way to begin is to respect one another. No matter how tired you get or how frustrated you feel, maintaining respect for each other helps any situation. Censor words that can hurt one another; speak as you would to a friend. Be nice in your interactions; kindness goes a long way.

Focus on what is important, and ignore extraneous elements. If you need help with a chore, ask for help, but don't go into detail about problems you are having in other areas. Save that for a time that you can sit down and talk in a relaxed way.

Compliment each other, whether it's about how the other one looks or about the fine job he or she is doing as a new parent. Everyone wants and needs to feel appreciated and loved, so remind each other again and again.

Thank your partner for what he or she does for you. "Thank you" is very powerful and affirming in any relationship. It also shows respect for what the other person is doing (or attempting to do).

Make time to hug and to kiss each other. This nonsexual touching is important in a relationship, especially when you may not have time for sex.

Set aside time every day for each other. Even if it's only 5 minutes at bedtime, knowing your partner is there for you (or you for him or her) with undivided attention can be very strengthening in a relationship. It stresses the importance of the bond between the two of you and maintains commitment and communication.

Get out together when you can. Try to arrange a time away from home and baby that allows the two of you to focus only on each other. It doesn't have to be a long time—a half-hour walk in the early evening while a neighbor watches the baby can help you reconnect with each other after days of hurry and rushing.

Laugh together. Life is serious but not all the time. Laughter heals, and it relieves tension. By laughing about various situations, you defuse them and relieve your tension. It's better to laugh than to cry, and it'll bring you closer together.

Listen, with respect when your partner wants to talk. It's important to help you stay connected. If you don't have time right then to talk, ask your partner to wait until you have the time to listen. Try to set a definite time to sit down to talk.

Admit that it's OK to have differences of opinion. Moms don't have all the answers; neither do dads. One of you may know more than the other, but that doesn't mean the other parent doesn't have valid points to make. It's often acceptable to do a chore or task in more than one way. You both could be right, so it's important to discuss a situation and come to an agreement. You might agree that you will each do the same task in different ways—or that you'll each do it *your own* way.

The importance of this section is to stress that closeness in your relationship can be maintained, even if your are both busy and stressed. It takes work, but it will pay off in many ways as you work together parenting your child.

Working Together as Parents

(For Both the New Mother and the New Father)

You'll probably find that if you begin your role as parents by working together, you'll accomplish a great deal more. Agree in the beginning that it's OK for each of you to have different ways of doing things, but that you will be consistent in whatever you do.

Consistency is one of the most-important aspects of raising a child. A child needs to know what the rules are and to have them consistently enforced. It's very confusing when the same action brings different reactions from each parent. If you set limits, stand by them all the time. It's hard to do, but your child will be much happier and better adjusted if you are consistent in your expectations, discipline and encouragement.

If you and your partner divide parenting duties and responsibilities as evenly as possible between the two of you, it will be easier for you to parent your baby. The fact that there are two of you will naturally introduce differences on the way some tasks should be handled, but this can be beneficial. Make an attempt to work together—not at odds with each other—to provide consistency in your child's life.

It's tough being a parent—it takes a lot of hard work, and it can be very stressful. But the rewards are great. Working together to create a team with your partner can increase those rewards.

One of the most-common areas of concern is disagreements—it will be impossible for you and your partner to agree on everything. It may help to understand that each of you will bring to this parenting relationship your own background of feelings and thoughts. You each may have a different "take" on a situation. This can create problems if you don't set up ways to deal with the differences in advance. The list below may provide you with some ways to deal with your particular situation.

Dealing with Your Differences

- Make plans before the baby arrives. Sit down and discuss what your expectations are before your baby is born. It's easier to find out what your partner believes is the way to parent before you each get caught up in the stress of parenting. You may be surprised (pleasantly or not) at what your partner believes his or her role as a parent will be.
- Make an effort to share duties. It's a good idea for each of you to know how to care for your child completely, not just to know how to perform certain tasks. Because of illness or a change in the family situation, roles may change. If you are both experienced in all facets of caring for your baby, you'll be able to handle any changes more easily.

- Agree what behaviors will or will not be tolerated. Establishing boundaries before a problem occurs provides direction for dealing with any future problems when they arise.
- Decide on a course of action to deal with a situation. Making this decision beforehand establishes a way to resolve a problem. If discipline is necessary as the child grows older, both parents know what is appropriate for the child.
- Stay flexible. Different people have different ways of doing things that bring the same results. There is usually a variety of solutions at hand—be open to doing things a different way. It may save time and effort on your part to accept the "different" way your partner does something.
- Support each other, even if you have a difference of opinion. Wait until you are alone to talk about your different responses to the situation, and work together to resolve it. Remain united in front of your child.
- Work toward an emotional balance. Support each other in your efforts to be good parents.

Consider each other's perspective. When a situation arises that you disagree on, try to see it from the other's point of view. Sometimes this shift in perspective can be very beneficial to you both.

Make Time for Each Other

(For Both the New Mother and the New Father)

With a new baby in the house, you may find you just don't seem to have time for each other like you used to. Sex may seem like a thing of the past. Sitting down and relating to one another as adults may seem like a luxury you can't indulge in any more. You used to spend time alone together, but now you just don't.

Your relationship as a couple is still very important. In fact, it is more important than ever because you really *need* your partner's love and support now more than ever before. Take heart. There are some things you can do for your partner and your relationship. It takes planning, work and time, but you'll be glad you did it when you reconnect.

You can make those spare minutes you have together count. All it takes is a little extra planning.

Tips to Help You Remain Connected to Your Partner

- Write yourself notes or leave yourself messages on your answering machine when you're out. They'll help remind you to make the time you need to be together, even when you get caught up in the hectic business of taking care of the baby.
- Arrange a babysitter for a short time. Ask family and friends to sit with the baby while you go out together. Exchange babysitting duties with another couple who has a new baby. You don't have to go out to a fancy restaurant or spend a lot of money. Just getting away and being alone together is what is most important.
- Splurge occasionally. For example, have a take-out restaurant deliver your dinner to your home to allow you extra time together.
- Make a "date" for home. Set aside time to be together, just the two of you. After you put the baby down, take the phone off the hook and just concentrate on each other. Watch a video together, or drink a glass of wine.
- Cut corners when and where you can. Let the laundry go for a while. Leave cleaning the kitchen till later. Devise shortcuts for doing chores and tasks.
- You don't have to be perfect. If your house isn't spotless, it's OK. Wouldn't you rather have a little dust on the tables and a more-solid relationship with your partner?
- Instead of doing tasks separately, do them together. Work on a project with your partner, like working in the garden or washing the car. Doing something together gets the job done in half the time, and you get to be with one another while you're doing it.
- Create time to be together. Try getting up a little earlier to share time. Call one another during the day to reconnect. Let other things slide a little, such as returning phone calls, so you can be together.

Paternity Leave

(For the New Father)

United States federal law guarantees a new father time to be at home with his baby, but few fathers take advantage of it. Many do not know much about the law. Others fear they might lose their job or be punished in some way if they request it. Below is some valuable information for you so you'll know more about paternity leave and can decide if it's for you.

Many men want to take time off from work after their child is born to get to know their baby better. They want to grow closer to their child, gain confidence in their parenting skills and become more comfortable as a parent.

The Family and Medical Leave Act of 1993 (FMLA) grants all workers (men and women) in companies with 50 or more employees up to 12 weeks' unpaid time off in the first year after a baby's birth to care for a baby. This act made millions of fathers eligible for paternity leave, but few have taken advantage of it. In fact, fewer than 20% of those who are eligible have actually taken time off.

Why haven't men taken paternity leave? Most have claimed that they can't afford to lose a paycheck. Others are afraid their bosses will think they aren't committed to their careers. Some fear that they will be fired from their jobs for taking the time off, even though the law guarantees protection against this occurrence.

It's important for you to know you *can* take unpaid leave after your baby's birth. Being able to stay at home with your child is a wonderful gift. As one father who stayed at home for 6 weeks with his new son said, "You can't believe how quickly they grow and change. The time with him made me realize I could do the job (of parenting) and do it well. I think we'll always be close because of the time we shared together. I wouldn't give this up for the world!"

CHAPTER 9

Returning to Work

Your pregnancy is over, and it seems as if most of the hard work is done. Yet you must still deal with a variety of issues, from what kind of childcare arrangement you choose to whether both you and your partner will work full time. You'll come to realize that balancing a family and a career requires organization and flexibility.

Whether to continue working outside the home after the baby's birth is one decision that many mothers wish they didn't have to make. However, due to financial necessity, not going back to work is not an option for many women.

In the 1950s and early 1960s, few women with children under the age of 6 worked outside the home. Today, a woman's salary may not be expendable. That's the reason more than half of all mothers (about 60%) work outside the home. Returning to work after having a baby is as common as staying home.

One major consideration that many couples do not take into account when the woman returns to work is the cost of working. It may surprise you how much it will cost when you return to work after giving birth. Below is a list to consider as you total the costs of working outside your home:

- cost of childcare
- cost of formula, if you are bottlefeeding
- cost of equipment that is duplicated between home and daycare

- the increase in taxes from a dual income
- costs of travel to and from work, including the extra time it will take you to take your child to daycare
- meals eaten at work (unless you bring your lunch)
- miscellaneous costs, such as dry cleaning, clothing, travel expenses
- any "treats" you reward yourself with because of the time and effort you have to put into your job, like eating out or buying convenience foods

To figure your hourly rate, add the amount you take home for each pay period to the value of your benefits. Deduct the total costs, then divide the number by the number of hours you spend away from home. You may be surprised by the bottom-line figure!

If You Decide to Stay at Home

You may decide to stay home with your baby. If you do, the change from going out each day to work to staying at home can be very dramatic. Studies have shown that some women who left full-time careers and did not return to work after their baby was born were more distressed than new mothers who returned to work! You may find that staying at home isn't as easy as you thought it would be—it's true won't have to worry about getting to work or coming home to fix meals and do housework, but you may find staying home means less companionship, less money and a loss of your daily work routine.

If you have worked full time, you may not have met many people in your area or neighborhood. It's hard to make friends when you work all day. Once you're home full time, you may be surprised at how many friends you'll make as a new mother. You'll find your neighborhood may become a substitute for your workplace. Be sure you don't bury yourself in motherhood and exclude all other activities. Make an effort to get out, meet people and get involved in new experiences with your baby.

It might be a good idea to stay in touch with your colleagues at work. Drop in to see them, or go out to lunch with a group. Call them, and stay on top of what is happening in your field.

Before You Return to Work

If you make the decision to return to work, there are some things you can do that will make the transition from home to career easier and more successful. These ideas come from women all over the world who have done it.

2 Weeks Before You Return to Work
It's important to experiment with various feeding techniques before you make any final decisions. You may decide to continue breastfeeding your baby. You can do this fairly easily if you are close to work or your job offers daycare services, allowing you to visit your baby when it's time to feed him. If these are not options, you will have to pump your breasts; use a dual-action pump to get the job done twice as fast. If you decide to switch to formula, eliminate one nursing every couple of days. It might help to begin with the early evening feeding. Switch to formula for day feedings. Eliminate the first and last feedings of the day as your final switch to formula.

Examine your wardrobe, and try clothes on! You may be larger in size (it's only natural), or your body shape may have changed somewhat, making some clothes fit differently. Be sure you try on shoes first. Many women find that their shoe size increases during pregnancy and often doesn't return to prepregnancy size after they have given birth. If you intend to breastfeed or pump your breasts during working hours, you may need clothes that allow you to do this easily.

Make sure daycare arrangements have been finalized. Visit the place you have planned to leave your child to check it out again and make sure they have enrolled your child.

It's a good idea to have alternate arrangements made, in case your child gets sick and you can't take her to daycare. If you use a babysitter, you may need an alternate sitter in case *she* gets sick.

Evaluate your needs at home. Will you be able to eliminate certain chores or adapt yourself to accept different standards? You may not realize how valuable your time will be when you are at home—you probably don't want to spend your time keeping everything sparkling. Can you do chores more efficiently, such as cooking ahead for the week or shopping only once a week?

1 Week Before You Return to Work
It may seem rather strange to do this, but begin your work routine this week. Get up at the same time you would normally if you were going to work. Feed your baby on the new schedule. Make and eat your own breakfast.

Make a list of all the supplies you will need for the baby at home and at daycare. Consider diapers, formula, baby clothes, extra bottles, a second car seat and anything that is particular for your baby's care and comfort.

On the night before you go back to work, choose your clothes, and make sure everything is OK to wear. Pack your diaper bag with everything your baby will need when you take her to daycare. Eat a good meal, and go to bed early to get a good night's sleep.

The Day You Return to Work
If possible, choose a Thursday to return to work. It will help you get into the routine of working, but as you will only work a very short week, it will allow you to replenish your energy for the following 5-day work week.

If you can start back with fewer hours, that will also help. Five hours a day for a week is a good plan, gradually increasing to 8 hours a day.

Plan easy-to-fix meals for the first few weeks after you start working. You might even want to get take-home food a couple of times.

Don't be upset with yourself if you feel a great loss when you return to work. It's OK to grieve and even feel some guilt when you leave your baby. You may even feel some relief to get back to work. That's OK, too.

If you continue to breastfeed, take extra clothing to work with you. Be sure you have a good supply of breast pads, too.

Going Back to Work

When you return to work, you'll find that some co-workers are very supportive; others may be insensitive to you and how you are feeling. It's important to find ways to ease the transition from being at home to going back to work.

You may encounter some of your greatest challenges when you return home after work. You'll be tired and hungry, but you probably won't be able to sit down and rest, as your family will need your time and attention. You may need to arrange with your partner to share many new "baby" responsibilities. Give your baby your total attention when you are with her. Have your partner try to do the same by having him spend some quality time with her. Set aside time for just you and your partner. You'll probably both need it after a full day.

It's important to manage your time; you'll have many new demands on you and your resources. Try to make a plan and stick to it. You can't do everything, so don't try. Delegate some responsibilities to others. Do what you can, and let less-important things go. You may not be able to do as much as you could before your baby was born; you may need to change your expectations.

Childcare Decisions

Arranging childcare can be a daunting task. There are many decisions you must make in selecting someone to care for your baby. Of course, you want to pick the best environment and caregiver for your child. The best way to do that is to know what your options are before you begin.

There are many choices when it comes to childcare. Any situation could be right for you, but you must first examine your needs and the needs of your child before you can decide which one to pursue. Below is a discussion of various types of childcare situations. Your options for childcare include:

- in-your-home care by a family relative
- in-your-home care by a nonrelative
- care in a caregiver's home
- a childcare center

In-home Care

You may decide on in-home care, either by a relative or nonrelative. Usually, having someone come to your home to take care of your child is much easier. You don't have to get the baby ready before you go in the morning, and you never have to take your child out in bad weather. It also takes less time in the morning and evening if you don't have to drop off or pick up your baby.

In-home care is an excellent choice for a baby or small child because it provides one-to-one attention if you only have one child at home. The environment is also familiar to the child.

When the caregiver is a relative, such as a grandparent, a sister or someone else in the family, you may find it more challenging than you anticipated. It may be more difficult to maintain your relationship with your caregiver while asking or telling him or her to do things the way you want them done.

When the caregiver is a nonrelative, you may find it very expensive to have this person come to your home. You are also hiring someone you do not know to come into your home and tend your child. You must be diligent in asking for references and checking them out thoroughly.

One drawback to having in-home care is the isolation your child may feel as he grows older. Children need to interact with other children so they can learn to share and play together. While in-home care can be an excellent choice for your baby, as he gets older you may have to make special arrangements to create opportunities for the child to be with other children.

Care in a Caregiver's Home

Taking your child to someone else's home is an option that many parents choose. Often these homes have small-group sizes that offer more flexibility for parents, such as keeping the child longer on a day when you may have a late meeting you cannot avoid. A homelike setting will make your child feel comfortable, and he may also receive lots of attention.

However, homes are not regulated in every state, so you must check out each situation very carefully. Contact your state's Department of Social Services, and ask about legal requirements. In some places, local agencies oversee caregivers who are members of their organization. Those who provide care must abide by certain standards, such as the maximum number of children allowed in the home (including their own), the maximum fees they may charge and attaining certain standards, such as CPR and first-aid certification.

Steps for Finding an In-home Caregiver

Whether you choose to have someone come to your home or to take your child to another person's home, there are some steps you can use to find a care provider. Following the steps listed below can help you find the best caregiver for your child.

Advertise in local newspapers and church bulletins to find someone to interview. Make sure you state how many children are to be cared for and their ages, and include information on the days and hours care is needed, the amount or type of experience you require and any other particulars. State that references will be required, and that these will be checked.

Talk to people on the telephone first to determine whether you want to interview them. Ask about their experience, qualifications, childcare philosophy and what they are seeking in a position. Then decide if you want to pursue the contact with an interview in person. Make a list of all your concerns, including the days and hours someone is needed, the duties to be performed, the need for a driver's license and what kind of benefits policy will be supplied. Discuss these with the potential caregiver.

Check all references. Have the potential caregiver provide you with the names and phone numbers of people he or she has worked for in the past. Call each of the families, let them know you are considering this person as a caregiver and discuss it with them.

Check it out. After you hire someone, monitor the situation occasionally by dropping by unannounced. See how everything is being managed when you do this. Pay attention to how your child reacts each time you leave or arrive; this can give you a clue as to how your child feels about the caregiver.

Responsibilities to Your Caregiver
As your caregiver has certain responsibilities to you, you have responsibilities to him or her. Be on time when you drop your child off or pick him up. Call if you're going to be late, even if the care is in your own home. Pay the caregiver when fees are due. Provide diapers, formula or expressed breast milk, extra clothes and personal items for the baby when necessary.

You must pay federal, state and local taxes for your care provider, including Social Security and Medicare taxes. If the person works in your home, you may also need to pay Workers' Compensation and unemployment insurance taxes. Contact the Internal Revenue Service and your state's Department of Economic Security for further information.

Childcare Centers

A childcare center is an environment in which many children are cared for in a larger setting. Centers vary widely in the facilities and activities they provide, the amount of attention they give each child, group sizes and childcare philosophy.

Inquire about the training required for each childcare provider or teacher. Some facilities expect more from a care provider than others. In some cases, a facility hires only trained, qualified personnel, or they train them and provide additional training.

You may find some childcare centers do not accept infants. Often centers focus more on older children; infants take a great deal of time and attention. If the center accepts infants, the ratio of caregivers to children should be about one adult to every three or four children (up to age 2). For older children, one adult for every four to six 2-year-olds and one adult for every seven to eight 3-year-olds is considered the maximum.

You want the facility you choose to offer quality childcare, but don't be fooled by a state-of-the-art center. Even the cleanest, brightest place is useless without the right kind of caregivers. Check out the center thoroughly; visit it by appointment, then stop in unannounced a few times. Meet the person in charge and the people who will care for your child. Ask for references from parents whose children are currently being cared for there. Call and talk to these parents before making a final decision.

Caring for an Infant

Babies have special needs that a preschool cannot provide for; be sure the place you choose for your infant can meet those needs. A baby must be changed and fed, but she also has other needs. A baby needs to be held and interacted with; she needs to be comforted when she is afraid. She needs to rest at certain times each day.

When searching for a place, keep in mind what will be required for your baby. Evaluate every situation according to whether it meets the needs of your baby.

Finding Childcare for Your Child

You might find it difficult to begin your search for someone to care for your child. Where do you start? There are many things you can do in your quest to find the best care situation for your child.

Ways to Find Out About Childcare

- Ask friends, family and co-workers for referrals to people or places they know about.
- Talk to people in your area.
- Ask at your church about any programs they may sponsor.
- Call a local referral agency, or contact Child Care Aware at 1-800-424-2246 for a local childcare resource.
- If you're interested in hiring a nanny to provide care in your home, contact a referral agency; they are usually listed in the yellow pages.

Whomever you choose to provide care for your child, *be sure* to check their references carefully before you make a final decision. This applies to centers as well as in-home caregivers (your home or theirs).

The Cost of Childcare

Paying for childcare can be a big-budget item in your household expenses. For some families, it can cost as much as 25% of their household budget.

The cost of infant and toddler care (through age 3) is the highest—it can range from $100 to $200 a week, depending on the type of care you choose. In-home care can be more costly, with placement fees and additional fees you negotiate based on extra tasks you want the caregiver to perform.

Public funding is available for some limited-income families. Title EE is a program paid for with federal funds. Call your local Department of Social Services to see if you are eligible.

Other programs to help in dealing with childcare costs include a federal tax-credit program, the dependent-care-assistance program and earned-income tax credit. These three programs are regulated by the federal government; contact the Internal Revenue service at 1–800–829–1040 for further information.

When to Start Looking for Childcare

Finding the best situation for your baby can take time. Start the process several weeks (maybe several months, particularly in special situations like twins) before you need it. Often this means finding childcare before your baby is born.

Some situations may require getting on a waiting list. There is a shortage of quality childcare for children under age 2. If you find a care provider you are comfortable with, but it's not time to leave your baby, ask if you can put down a deposit and set a date for childcare to begin. Keep in touch with the care provider, and plan to meet before you place your child in daily care.

Special-Care Needs

In some situations, your child may have special-care needs. If your baby is born with a disability or a health problem that needs one-on-one attention, you may have a harder time finding appropriately qualified childcare. In these special cases, you may have to spend extra time seeking a suitably qualified care provider.

Contact the hospital where your child has been cared for and ask for references, or contact your pediatrician. They may be in contact with someone who can help you. It may be better if you have a child with special needs to arrange for a care provider to come to your home.

Caring for a Sick Child

All children come down with colds, the flu or diarrhea at some time. Today, there are ways to deal with your child's illness if you can't take time off from work to stay at home with him.

In many places, "sick-child" daycare centers are available. They are usually attached to a regular daycare facility, although some are connected with hospitals. A sick-child center provides a comfortable place where a child who is ill can rest or participate in quiet activities, such as story time.

This kind of facility is often headed by a registered nurse who can administer medication when necessary. Fees for this type of service run from $25 to $55 a day.

Some cities have "on-call" in-home care providers who come to your home when your child is too sick to be taken anywhere. The program is usually run by an agency that deals with childcare, and these caregivers normally charge by the hour. Getting a person to come to your home is usually on a first-come, first-served basis, so you may have to wait a day for a provider. However, this can be an excellent way to care for a child who is too ill to be taken away from home.

Can You Modify Your Work Situation?

With careful exploration, there may be ways to modify your current work situation so everyone is happy—you, your boss, your partner and your baby. Various work schedules may be used to suit your needs.

Some women decide to keep working, but not full time. If there is some way you can cut your hours and work part time, you may be happier. It may mean less money, but your peace of mind may compensate for the monetary loss.

Ask your employer if you can cut your hours or share a job with someone else. There may be another person in the company who would like to work only part time.

Find out if flex-time programs are available at your workplace. In some cases, you can modify your work schedule; for example, you could work four 10-hour days. In other cases, you may be able to come in early and leave early, or arrive late and leave later. You may be able to set your own schedule, as long as you get your work done.

If you do work part time or flex-time, childcare may be harder to find. Some centers are more flexible than others, and some in-home care providers (their home or yours) welcome the break. In other cases, you may find less flexibility with a center—you usually pay on a weekly basis, whether your child is there or not. If an in-home care provider depends on the income from tending your child, a lighter schedule means less money.

A third solution might be to work at home part of the time or full time. If you work with a computer, many companies are now set up to allow workers (men and women) to do their computer work at home, while they are connected by modem to the company's computer. Working from home can be a positive experience for you and your baby.

Breastfeeding and Work

Breastfeeding is important to many women, and they don't want to have to stop when they return to work. You *don't* have to stop—it is possible to breastfeed even after you return to work. If you breastfeed exclusively, you will have to pump your breasts or arrange to see your baby during the day. Or you can nurse your baby at home and feed expressed breast milk or formula when you're away. It takes a little more time, but if it's important to you, do it. (See Chapter 4 for an in-depth discussion of breastfeeding.)

One way to smooth the back-to-work transition for you and baby is to begin storing breast milk for a couple of weeks before you return to work. Use an electric breast pump to express milk between feedings about 2 weeks before you start work. Don't start expressing milk sooner because you may produce too much milk. A breast pump that has a double-pumping feature empties both breasts at once.

Freeze expressed milk in quantities from 1 ounce to 4 ounces. This provides your caregiver with options as to how much to thaw for a particular feeding.

It may be possible to pump then store breast milk while you are at work. You may be very uncomfortable if you don't pump your breasts because your milk continues to flow in. Take a breast pump with you, and refrigerate or discard breast milk after it is pumped.

If you remain at home until your baby is between 4 and 6 months old, your baby may be able to skip the bottle and start drinking from a cup. Earlier than 4 months, your baby will need to learn to drink from a bottle. After 4 weeks of nursing only, your baby will be ready to try a bottle without compromising your milk supply or his nursing technique. With the first bottle feedings, let someone else feed the baby the bottle when he's not too hungry. Bottlefeed him around the same time he will receive a bottle once you return to work.

CHAPTER 10

Planning and Preparing for Your Next Pregnancy

It may seem strange to discuss your next pregnancy when you've just had a baby, but it's an important consideration. Most women want to wait for a while after they have had a baby before even thinking about pregnancy again, but some women want to get pregnant again very quickly. Other women are surprised when they find themselves pregnant again because they didn't think about birth control. Below is a discussion of many aspects of postpregnancy that you may not have thought about.

Your 6-Week Postpartum Checkup

Your 6-week postpartum checkup is a good time to ask questions about future pregnancies. Discuss your concerns or any complications that arose during your recent delivery. This information can be especially helpful if you relocate or plan to deliver with a different doctor or hospital in the future. Some common concerns include those listed below.

Common Concerns About Future Pregnancies

- Are there things you need to do before getting pregnant again?
- Are there any warning signs to watch out for during subsequent pregnancies?
- Were there complications during your last pregnancy that may recur, such as gestational diabetes?
- If you had a C-section, will you need to have one again next time or could you safely try labor?

Women frequently ask, "How long should I wait before getting pregnant again?" Another common question is, "Is there a difference in recovery between a vaginal delivery or a C-section, as far as future pregnancies are concerned?" A general answer is that you should first recover physically and emotionally before attempting pregnancy again, regardless of the type of delivery (C-section or vaginal delivery). How long your recovery takes is influenced by several factors, including the following:

- complications during your previous pregnancy, such as high blood pressure
- how long or difficult labor and delivery were
- problems with bleeding or infection
- medical problems, such as diabetes
- how much help you get at home from friends or family
- what responsibilities you already have at home (how many children and how old they are)

When we speak of *physical recovery*, we mean when you are able to do all the normal activities that you did before your pregnancy, when you have resumed regular exercise, when your weight is satisfactory, and when there are no medical or physical problems requiring tests or treatments that should be checked out before becoming pregnant again. For most women, this is at least 6 months to 1 year after delivery, at the earliest.

These guidelines are for recovery after a vaginal or a Cesarean delivery. Recovery from a C-section usually takes longer than recovery from a vaginal delivery. The main difference is the incision on your abdomen and the pain or discomfort that can make it a little harder to exercise or resume your normal activities as quickly as after a vaginal delivery.

Contraception Issues

Your 6-week postpartum checkup is a good time to talk to your doctor about your contraception plans for the future. Not every woman will be ready to resume relations; it's a very individual thing. It's a good idea to decide what to do for contraception at this point so that when you resume relations, you will have reliable contraception. We have known of a few women who had delivered two children in 1 year, and they were not twins!

Your decision on birth control can be affected by several factors. The options for those who are breastfeeding are a little different from those who are bottlefeeding.

Contraception Choices for Breastfeeding Moms

Breastfeeding protects you against getting pregnant for a while, but if you don't want a surprise, you should consider using some kind of contraception. At her first prenatal visit, Trish was asked the date of her last period (to determine a due date and how far along she was). When she answered, "15 months ago," it became clear that she hadn't had a more-recent period because for the last 15 months she had been either pregnant, or nursing the baby she had delivered 6 months ago. Her pregnancy actually occurred while she was nursing her baby!

Contraception choices for a nursing mom include:

- barrier methods, such as a condom or diaphragm
- spermicides in the form of gels or suppositories
- birth-control pills, called *minipills* (they contain the hormone *progesterone*, and are safe for a nursing mom and her baby)
- Depo-Provera®, a hormone injection given every 3 months
- an IUD (intrauterine device)
- Norplant®, small rods containing a hormone (progesterone) placed in the arm just under the skin

You should realize that while it is true that nursing can protect you from getting pregnant, you are living dangerously if you are not using another method while breastfeeding. Most women don't have periods while they are nursing during the first 6 months. But you could ovulate and get pregnant the longer you nurse; it's a mistake to think that not having a period means you are unable to get pregnant!

Contraception Choices for Bottlefeeding Moms

Contraceptive choices for the bottlefeeding mom are the same as those listed above, with one small exception. If you bottlefeed, regular birth-control pills should be used rather than the minipill, if you choose birth-control pills for contraception.

Pregnancy within the First Year

Most doctors recommend that you try to avoid getting pregnant again for at least 1 year after your delivery because during this time, you will be extremely busy with your new baby. You will have enough on your hands in learning to adjust to your new life while still finding time for yourself.

If you had any problems or complications during or after your pregnancy, be sure to take care of them so that when you do get pregnant again, you will be in the best possible health. If you take any medications on a regular basis, talk with your doctor before stopping or changing them, and find out if they can potentially harm a developing fetus. Usually, it is best to decrease the amount of medication you are taking, if possible, and to avoid or to stop taking any medications you don't need or that may be harmful to you and your developing baby. Let your doctor help you with this.

Women are frequently anxious to know if there is an exact time interval that is safe before trying to get pregnant again after a delivery. "How many months before I will know it's safe to start trying to get pregnant again?" The answer to this question is different for every woman, but there are some general guidelines. Whether you had an easy first pregnancy and delivery doesn't usually help to predict what will happen in subsequent pregnancies. Each pregnancy tends to be unique; don't count on future pregnancies being either easier or harder than your first one.

A couple also needs to recover physically and emotionally from the many changes and challenges introduced by their newborn. Recovering physically may take 6 months, a year or even longer. Part of this challenge is the full-time "job" required in caring for a newborn—it doesn't leave a lot of time for you. It may help to trade childcare with a friend in order to get time for exercise, time alone together as a couple or other personal time.

Many women are able to lose most, but not all, of the weight gained during a previous pregnancy. With each new pregnancy, some start out 5 to 10 pounds heavier than their prepregnancy weight. During each subsequent pregnancy, it can be even harder to control your weight; after two or three pregnancies, you will have gained 10 to 20 pounds that can be very hard to lose.

If you had any complications during this first pregnancy, labor or delivery, discuss them with your doctor. Find out what to watch for as you recover and if any complications during this pregnancy could affect another pregnancy. Most complications, such as anemia or gestational diabetes, begin to improve after delivery, and nothing more will need to be done. Some problems, such as high blood pressure, need to be re-evaluated after you have delivered. Make sure you check out any possible problems; have any necessary medical tests before attempting another pregnancy.

If you had a Cesarean (C-section), it may be necessary to deliver by C-section again. You could have a *trial of labor* (TOL), sometimes called a VBAC (*vaginal birth after C-section*).

If you had gestational diabetes last time, investigate whether this might be a problem next time. Whatever your concerns following your first delivery, it is best to discuss them with your doctor while they are fresh in both your minds. The answers to your questions about your recent pregnancy could make a big difference in preparing for any future pregnancy.

Make sure you take all of these things into consideration, and take whatever action is necessary before stopping contraception. (You may not think that you are trying to get pregnant, but if you are not using contraception, you are trying to get pregnant!) Today, it is becoming more common to refer to the "*12 months*" of pregnancy, rather than 9 months, meaning that you should begin treating yourself as though you are already pregnant 3 months *before* you actually do get pregnant.

You may wish to read the other pregnancy books in this series, *Your Pregnancy Questions & Answers, Your Pregnancy Week by Week* and *Your Pregnancy After 30*, for information on preparing for pregnancy. Reading them can be very helpful in your prepregnancy preparations, even if you have been pregnant before.

Whether you decide to have another baby in a year or two, or to wait a longer period of time, it's important to be prepared for your next pregnancy. By reading this book, so recovery from your last pregnancy is as complete as you can make it, and by taking the best care of yourself if you decide to become pregnant again, you'll go a long way to ensuring the good health of yourself and your next baby.

Glossary

anti-inflammatory medications Drugs to relieve pain or inflammation.

areola Pigmented area surrounding the nipple of the breast.

bilirubin Breakdown product of pigment formed in the liver from hemoglobin during the destruction of red blood cells.

board certification Doctor has had additional training and testing in a particular speciality. In the area of obstetrics, the American College of Obstetricians and Gynecologists offers this training. Certification requires expertise in care of a pregnant woman.

bonding Process in which a parent becomes emotionally attached to her or his child.

breast pump Hand, battery or electrically operated device used for expressing milk from the breast.

catheter Tubular device for insertion into canals, vessels, passageways or body cavities, usually to permit injection or withdrawal of fluid or to keep a passage open.

cervix Narrow outer end of the uterus.

Cesarean section (delivery) (Also called *C-section*.) Delivery of a baby through an abdominal incision rather than through the vagina.

chloasma Extensive brown patches of irregular shape and size on the face or other parts of the body.

circumcision Act of cutting off the foreskin (on a male).

colic Abdominal pain often caused by spasm, obstruction or twisting, which may be marked in a baby by episodes of loud, sudden crying and fussiness.

colostrum Thin, yellow fluid, which is the first milk to come from the breast.

Most often seen toward the end of pregnancy. It is different in content from milk produced later during nursing.

D & C (dilatation and curettage) Surgical procedure in which the cervix is dilated and the lining of the uterus is scraped.

DHA (Decosahexanoic acid.) Present in breast milk; forms the primary structural fatty acid that makes up the retina of the eye and the gray matter of the brain.

diaphragm Molded cap, usually of thin rubber, fitted over the cervix to act as a contraceptive barrier.

edema Swelling of tissues.

enema Fluid injected into the rectum for the purpose of clearing out the bowel.

engorgement Congested; filled with fluid.

epidural block Type of anesthesia. Medication is injected around the spinal cord during labor or other types of surgery.

episiotomy Surgical incision of the perineum (area between the vagina and the rectum). Used during delivery to avoid tearing or laceration of the vaginal opening and rectum.

gestational diabetes Occurrence or worsening of diabetes during pregnancy (gestation).

hemorrhoids Dilated blood vessels in the rectum or rectal canal.

HMO (Also called *health maintenance organization.*) Organization that provides comprehensive health care to enrolled individuals and families in a particular geographical area by member physicians. Financed by periodic payments determined in advance.

hypertension, pregnancy-induced High blood pressure that occurs during pregnancy. Defined by an increase in the diastolic and/or systolic blood pressure.

insulin Peptide hormone made by the pancreas. It promotes the use of glucose.

involution Shrinkage of the uterus after birth.

isoimmunization Development of specific antibody directed at the red blood cells of another individual, such as a baby *in utero*. Often occurs when an Rh-negative woman carries an Rh-positive baby or is given Rh-positive blood.

isometric exercise Exercise that pits one muscle or part of the body against another or against an immovable object.

isotonic exercise Exercise that tenses the muscles against a heavy or resistant force, helping to build up muscle strength.

IUD Interuterine device used for contraception.

I.V. Apparatus used to administer an intravenous injection or feeding; also, such an injection or feeding.

jaundice Yellow staining of the skin, sclera (eyes) and deeper tissues of the body. Caused by excessive amounts of bilirubin. Treated with phototherapy.

labor Process of expelling a fetus from the uterus.

linea nigra Line of increased pigmentation running down the abdomen from the bellybutton to the pubic area during pregnancy.

lochia Discharge of blood as the lining of the uterus is shed.

lymphoma Tumor of the lymphoid tissue.

mask of pregnancy Increased pigmentation over the area of the face under each eye.

menstruation Regular or periodic discharge of a bloody fluid from the uterus.

milk letdown Flow of milk into the breast ducts, usually occurring several times during breastfeeding. May also occur when woman hears a baby cry.

obstetrician Physician who specializes in the care of pregnant women and developing fetuses.

oral contraceptives Birth-control pills.

ovulation Cyclic production of an egg from the ovary.

oxytocin Hormone that causes the uterus to contract and breast milk to flow.

Pap smear Routine screening test that evaluates the presence of premalignant or cancerous conditions of the cervix.

perineum The area between the vagina and anus (rectum).

postpartum Pertaining to the period after birth.

postpartum blues Mild depression after delivery.

postpartum distress A range of symptoms including the baby blues, postpartum depression and postpartum psychosis. ·

postpartum hemorrhage A loss of more than 17 fluid ounces (500 ml) in the first 24 hours after delivery.

pre-eclampsia Combination of symptoms significant to pregnancy, including high blood pressure, protein in urine, swelling and changes in reflexes.

pregnancy diabetes See *gestational diabetes.*

premature delivery Delivery before 38 weeks gestation.

projectile vomiting Vomiting in which stomach contents are ejected with great force.

proteinuria Protein in urine.

Rh-negative Absence of rhesus antibody in the blood.

RhoGAM® Medication given during pregnancy and following delivery to prevent isoimmunization. See *isoimmunization.*

SIDS Sudden-infant-death syndrome.

sitz tub A chair-type bath, which soaks the thighs and hips.

skin tag Flap or extra buildup of skin.

sodium Element found in many foods, particularly salt. Ingestion of too much sodium may cause fluid retention.

spinal headache Type of headache that may be caused by an epidural or spinal anesthetic.

stretch marks Scars where skin has stretched due to enlarging abdomen and weight gained during pregnancy.

superficial thrombophlebitis Inflammation of the vein with formation of a blood clot.

tubal ligation Form of surgical sterilization that involves tying a woman's Fallopian tubes to prevent further pregnancies.

umbilical cord Cord that connects the placenta to the developing baby. It removes waste products and carbon dioxide from the baby and brings oxygenated blood and nutrients from the mother through the placenta to the baby.

urinary incontinence Problems controlling the flow of urine.

uterus (Also called a *womb*.) Organ an embryo/fetus grows in.

varicositites (Also called *varicose veins*.) Abnormally swollen or dilated veins.

vernix White or yellowy waxy substance that may cover part of a newborn's body.

Index